UNDERSTANDING
ARTHRITIS

UNDERSTANDING
ARTHRITIS

ARTHRITIS FOUNDATION

EDITOR:
Irving Kushner, M.D.

ASSOCIATE EDITORS:
Ann Forer and Ann B. McGuire

CHARLES SCRIBNER'S SONS · NEW YORK

Charles Scribner's Sons
Macmillan Publishing Company
866 Third Avenue, New York, N.Y. 10022
Collier Macmillan Canada, Inc.

Library of Congress Cataloging in Publication Data

Main entry under title:

Understanding arthritis.

  Bibliography: p.
  Includes index.
  1. Arthritis.   I. Kushner, Irving, 1929–
II. Arthritis Foundation.
RC933.U47   1985   616.7'22   82-22921
ISBN 0-684-18199-1
0-684-18736-1 (pbk.)

Macmillan books are available at special discounts for bulk purchases for sales promotions, premiums, fund-raising, or educational use. For details, contact:

  Special Sales Director
  Macmillan Publishing Company
  866 Third Avenue
  New York, N.Y. 10022

Also available in hardcover from Charles Scribner's Sons

10 9 8 7 6 5

Printed in the United States of America

This book is not intended as a substitute for the medical advice of physicians. The reader should regularly consult a physician in matters relating to his or her health and particularly in respect of any symptoms which may require diagnosis or medical attention.

Contents

Contents

Acknowledgments
and Contributors:
How This Book Came About

This book grew out of the efforts of the Arthritis Foundation's Public Education Committee, and is an expansion of a successful series of pamphlets on rheumatic diseases. The ongoing series began when volunteer rheumatologists provided the Public Education Committee with drafts of individual pamphlets, which the Arthritis Foundation staff then edited for lay readers and distributed through the local chapters of the Arthritis Foundation. During this process, the Public Education Committee became interested in making the information more readily available through libraries and bookstores, in a format that could serve as a general reference on arthritis. This interest coincided with that of Charles Scribner's Sons to publish a health book on arthritis.

This book would not have been possible without the cooperation of numerous people volunteering their time and expertise. The group of distinguished rheumatologists who provided much of the material for Part II, the chapters on individual rheumatic diseases, consist of Andrei Calin, M.D.; Rene Caillet, M.D.; John J. Calabro, M.D.; Edmund L. Dubois, M.D.; George E. Ehrlich, M.D.; Denys K. Ford, M.D.; Louis A. Healey, M.D.; P. Kahler Hench, M.D.; E. Carwile Leroy, M.D.; Roland W. Moscowitz, M.D.; Carl M. Pearson, M.D.; Paul G. Rochmis, M.D.; Jane G. Schaller, M.D.; Frank R. Schmid, M.D.; H. Ralph Schumacher, M.D.; and Kenneth R. Wilske, M.D. Mavis B. Cox also contributed to the chapter on systemic lupus erythematosus.

A second group of leaders in rheumatology also gave of their time, providing valuable insights into research developments and the basic disease processes involved in the course of rheumatic diseases. They are John Baum, M.D.; Rodney Bluestone, M.B., F.R.C.P.; Kenneth D. Brandt, M.D.; Charles L. Christian, M.D.; William E. Crowe, M.D.; Herbert S. Diamond, M.D.; James F. Fries, M.D.; Allan Gibofsky, M.D.; Robert A. Greenwald, M.D.; Maria Guttadauria, M.D.; Alan A. Halpern, M.D.; David S. Howell, M.D.; Joeseph E. Levinson, M.D.; Hildegard R. Maricq, M.D.; Daniel J. McCarty, M.D.; Thomas A. Medsger, Jr., M.D.; Paul E. Phillips, M.D.; Gerald P. Rodnan, M.D.; Peter H. Schur, M.D.; Peter Stastny, M.D.; Cody K. Wasner, M.D.; and Gerald Weissmann, M.D. Also, E. Y. Chao provided valuable information regarding bioengineering and joint replacement surgery.

Mr. Charles C. Bennett, former vice president for Public Education, had a major role in the early stages of organizing this project. The editor, Irving Kushner, M.D., was assisted in the process of organizing the pamphlet material into book form by Ann Forer and Ann B. McGuire. Frederic C. McDuffie, M.D., senior vice president for Medical Affairs, contributed to the final review process preceding publication.

THE ARTHRITIS FOUNDATION

About the Editors

IRVING KUSHNER, M.D., is Professor of Medicine at Case Western Reserve University in Cleveland, and Director of the Division of Rheumatology at Cleveland Metropolitan General/ Highland View Hospital. He is also Associate Director of the hospital's Department of Medicine. Dr. Kushner has long been a member of the American Rheumatism Association and has been President of its Central Region. He has served on many Arthritis Foundation and American Rheumatism Association committees, including the Committee on Public Education, and he was chairman of the Foundation's Review Panel for Medical and Scientific Publications. Dr. Kushner is a graduate of Columbia University, New York, and Washington University School of Medicine, St. Louis, Missouri.

ANN FORER has been writing about health and medicine for more than a decade, interpreting developments in medical research and clinical practice for the consumer. Her work has appeared in magazines, books, pamphlets, and on television and has been the basis of educational films. She is a specialist in arthritis, genetics, and birth defects. She was formerly Associate Director of Public Information for the Arthritis Foundation and served on its Committee on Public Education. She was also Associate Editor at the March of Dimes Birth Defects Foundation and Vice President of Manning, Selvage and Lee in New York City, where she directed programs in science and medicine information. She presently lives in Montclair, New Jersey.

ANN B. MCGUIRE is currently Managing Editor for Professional Publications at the Arthritis Foundation and was previously Medical Writer for the Foundation. Among other publications, she is responsible for the bimonthly *Bulletin on the Rheumatic Diseases*. She has a degree in biology from the University of California, Santa Cruz, with an emphasis in science writing and previously served as Science Editor for the University of California, Davis.

Introduction

Arthritis is a very common ailment (one out of every seven Americans has it), yet is vastly misunderstood. It is the subject of an abundant folklore, many half-truths, and a thriving quackery business. Many people are surprised to learn that the term "arthritis" actually refers to more than one hundred different diseases. Many are also unaware that arthritis can affect people at any age—not just older people—and that it can be very serious. Perhaps the most harmful popular belief is the notion that nothing can be done for someone in whom arthritis appears. To the contrary, prompt and continuing treatment can bring many forms of this disease under control.

Strictly speaking, the word "arthritis" means joint inflammation (from the Greek "arth" meaning joint, and "itis" meaning inflammation). This inflammation is not a single disease itself, but rather a feature of many related diseases that can affect the different joints and parts of the body. As a group, these diseases are referred to as the rheumatic diseases. Besides the joints, these diseases can also affect the skin, the tissues surrounding the joints, the muscles, and virtually every organ in the body. Many people easily recognize joint inflammation—the pain, swelling, redness, and stiffness that often come with a rheumatic disease—but do not always know that it may signify a serious disease requiring medical attention.

Fortunately, most people who develop arthritis can continue to lead productive lives—if they see a qualified doctor soon after noticing the warning signs, follow their treatment plans closely, and keep a positive outlook on life.

Unfortunately, many bookstores, newspapers, television programs, and magazines are chock-full of misinformation about arthritis. So, too, are the well-meaning friends and family members of many people who develop arthritis. Moreover, much of the advertising for pain-relieving products encourages people to believe that arthritis of any type is nothing more than a group of "minor aches and pains." Quackery continues to flourish, in the form of false claims for quick "cures" and denouncements of the medical profession for allegedly ignoring the great number of people who have arthritis.

The truth is that remarkable progress has recently been made in fighting the effects of the rheumatic diseases. Early recognition and control of the different forms of these diseases have resulted in far fewer people developing serious joint deformities than did only a few decades ago. New information has begun to clarify the complex ways in which these diseases harm the body, and has led to the development of new drugs that often reduce that harm. Research and experience have shown that there are ways in which people with rheumatic disease can learn to protect their damaged joints from added stress. Therapeutic exercise programs can help such people to keep their joints working as well as possible, and they can also be taught effective ways of coping with arthritis and learn how their emotions affect their disease.

The problem is that too few members of the public—and especially those who would benefit the most from it—are aware of this progress. Overcoming arthritis requires each person to follow a broad treatment program tailored to his or her condition. To do this effectively, the person must learn as much as possible about that specific condition and the reasoning behind each aspect of its treatment.

The major purpose of this book is to provide accurate information to those who have arthritis, and to their concerned families and friends. It can also serve as a general reference for interested students, members of the media, and employers seeking answers to the problems that arthritis can pose in the workplace.

The two sections of the book complement each other. Section I provides a general overview of arthritis: of what may occur in the body when this condition develops, of both the accepted treatments and unproven remedies for it, and of ways of coping with its emotional and financial effects. Section II focuses on the sixteen most common forms of rheumatic disease. For ease of reading, each of the medical terms in the book is defined when it is first used, and a glossary of these terms is included at the back of the book.

Throughout this book you will find references to various aids that can help the person with arthritis live more comfortably. A complete description of such aids and the addresses of suppliers are listed in the *Self-Help Manual for Patients with Arthritis,* available through local chapters of the Arthritis Foundation for a nominal fee.

If you have arthritis, you need information. This book can help you understand what is happening in your body, learn to accept and live productively wth your condition, and raise questions that you will want to ask your doctor. It is not meant to take the place of proper medical treatment, but to encourage you to become involved in your own care. As you read through it, you will realize that you can learn how to control your arthritis, rather than sit back and let it control you.

PART ONE

GENERAL PRINCIPLES
ABOUT ARTHRITIS

CHAPTER ONE

An Overview of Arthritis

Arthritis is a major national health problem, one that affects people of all ages, races, geographical areas, and socioeconomic levels, and of both sexes. According to the 1980 Health Interview Survey by the U.S. Public Health Service, an estimated 37 million Americans have arthritis. Approximately one in seven Americans and one in three families are affected with one kind of arthritis or another. These estimates include many children. In fact, almost everyone who lives long enough will develop some joint damage from years of wear and tear and minor injuries to the joints.

The various forms of arthritis put a significant drain on the national economy and on individual pocketbooks: the condition costs our country more than $13 billion every year, a number that is broken down in Table 1. These costs do not even begin to reflect the emotional or physical tolls paid by people who have one of the rheumatic diseases or by their families. The table also does not include other costs, such as those of disability payments to people whose arthritis has made them unable to work for a living.

Most of the figures reported in Table 1 are based on statistics from government surveys done in 1975. We have translated these statistics into 1983 numbers by adjusting for higher costs to consumers and the increased number of people who now have arthritis. In Table 1, under Indirect Costs, "institutionalized people" refers to those who have been placed in hospitals, nursing homes, or other extended-care facilities because of arthritis;

Table 1: SOME ECONOMIC COSTS OF ARTHRITIS*

Direct Costs of Medical Care, Annual

Hospitalization	$ 1,431,000,000
Physician visits	1,238,000,000
Services from other health professionals	322,000,000
Drugs	798,000,000
Nursing home care	679,000,000
Unproven remedies	1,758,000,000
TOTAL, direct	$ 6,226,000,000

Indirect Costs of Medical Care, Annual

Lost wages	$ 6,046,000,000
Lost homemaker services	661,000,000
Lost wages and homemaker services for institutionalized people	239,000,000
Earnings lost due to early death	97,000,000
TOTAL, indirect	$ 7,043,000,000

TOTAL ANNUAL ECONOMIC COSTS	$13,269,000,000

* Extrapolated for 1982 costs from National Center for Health Statistics' Health Interview Survey, Nursing Home Survey, and Hospital Discharge Survey, 1975.

their lost wages and homemaker services are estimated from their expected earnings if they did not have arthritis.

SOME MAJOR FORMS OF ARTHRITIS

As mentioned in the Introduction to this book, "arthritis" literally means "joint inflammation," but is a feature of many different rheumatic diseases. Although these diseases have some aspects in common, each has its own pattern of symptoms and range of possible treatments. Most rheumatic diseases are chronic; that is, they often last a long time or recur many times throughout a person's life. Most forms have no cure. Their symptoms commonly come and go without warning. Those periods during which the disease causes no symptoms are called remissions; the times when the disease is active are termed flare-ups. Remissions and flare-ups can last from a few days to many years. Even during long remissions, however, treatment programs often must be continued to prevent or reduce later flare-ups.

Despite their similarities, the various forms of arthritis have distinct differences. This point can be underscored with a brief look at the features of some of the major rheumatic diseases. These diseases include osteoarthritis, rheumatoid arthritis, systemic lupus erythematosus (also known as lupus or SLE), ankylosing spondylitis, and gout.

Osteoarthritis, the most common kind of arthritis involves the breakdown of cartilage and sometimes bone. It is frequently mild but can become severe. Osteoarthritis is often considered to be the result of years of normal wear and tear on joints, but can also develop after damage to a joint from injury or infection. Although the disease can affect any joint, the ones most commonly involved are those of the fingers, and the hips, knees, and spine. Usually, only a few joints are affected.

Rheumatoid arthritis is potentially a very serious form of arthritis and may lead to severe joint deformity. It involves a chronic inflammation that can attack not only joints but also the skin, muscles, and blood vessels, and in rare cases, the lungs and heart. The pain, stiffness, swelling, and other effects of the disease flare up unpredictably, often affecting many joints and causing general whole-body illness as well as damage to the joint tissues.

Systemic lupus erythematosus affects many more women than men, and can damage the skin, joints, and internal organs, such as the kidneys. At one time, it was a very serious, often fatal disease, but early diagnosis and treatment have now enabled most people with systemic lupus to live nearly normal lives. There is no set pattern of symptoms at the beginning, and people with this disease sometimes go for several years before their doctors can diagnose it as lupus. Joint swelling and pain may or may not be present, but if they are, they usually do not produce permanent damage or crippling.

Ankylosing spondylitis is a kind of arthritis that affects the spine. As a result of inflammation, the bones of the spine fuse, or grow together. Many people with this disease are not seriously limited by it, but some have moderately active or severe spondylitis that restricts free movement of their backs and necks. Spondylitis can also affect the shoulders, knees, and ankles, as well as the eyes, heart, and lungs.

Gout is an acutely painful form of arthritis and is far more common than most people think, affecting about one million Americans. It results from a chemical defect that allows too much uric acid to build up in the body. Gout attacks occur when the uric acid forms crystals that become lodged in a joint —frequently the big toe—causing inflammation. Gout affects far more men than it does women.

It is important to understand that the term "chronic," as applied to the rheumatic diseases, does not mean hopeless. Recent advances in treating these diseases have allowed many people to continue to live comfortably and to reduce their risks of developing serious joint damage. Moreover, treatment for the rheumatic diseases has today become much more specific than it was in the past, being tailored for the specific disease and individual involved. It consists of far more than simply taking drugs, and may include special exercises, the use of devices to protect the joints, rest periods balanced with periods of activity, counseling, methods for controlling pain, the safe use of affected joints, and sometimes—if damage or pain has become severe— surgery to repair or replace damaged joints.

Still, designing treatments for rheumatic disease has not become an exact science. Some programs work better for some people than for others. For this reason, doctors often require a trial period for each person with such a disease, during which they prescribe different drugs and combinations of treatments to see how that person responds. But even though different people may respond differently to the same treatment, the sooner treatment is begun after any kind of arthritis has developed, the more likely it is to be successful. Unfortunately, people with arthritis do not always seek medical care promptly; most wait an average of four years after their symptoms first appear before getting medical help. During this time, their disease may cause permanent joint damage that could have been reduced or avoided with early treatment.

How does someone know when to seek medical care for aches and pains? If they know the arthritis warning signs, they'll be ready to act at the right time.

ARTHRITIS WARNING SIGNS

- Swelling in one or more joints
- Early-morning stiffness
- Recurring pain or tenderness in any joint
- Inability to move a joint normally
- Obvious redness and warmth in a joint
- Unexplained weight loss, fever, or weakness combined with joint pain
- Symptoms like these persisting for more than two weeks

If you have two or more of these signs, it is time to see a doctor for a diagnosis and proper treatment. It is also important to encourage someone who is experiencing several of these signs to seek qualified medical care.

THE TREATMENT TEAM

Many people wonder which kind of doctor is best suited to treat someone with arthritis. Usually, your family doctor is the right one to see at first. Your family physician is ordinarily aware of your overall health, the medications you take, past injuries that could affect your arthritis, and possible effects your job or lifestyle may have on the disease. Anyone without a family doctor can get help in finding one by calling the local county medical association.

For most people with arthritis, the family doctor will continue to provide ongoing care, but sometimes medical care by a specialist is also necessary. For a difficult diagnosis or treatment of the more serious kinds of arthritis, your family doctor may refer you to a rheumatologist, a physician who specializes in the rheumatic diseases. Depending on the disease and your condition, the rheumatologist may provide continuing care or design a treatment program for you to follow under the guidance of your family doctor. If surgery becomes a possibility, you will need to see an orthopedic surgeon (a doctor specializing in bone surgery) or a surgeon who specializes in hand surgery (usually an orthopedic or plastic surgeon). In

7

other situations, you may be referred to a physiatrist, a doctor specializing in physical medicine and rehabilitation.

The family physician or rheumatologist may at times refer the person with arthritis to other health professionals who have had special training and experience in treating this condition. These professionals include nurses, physical therapists, occupational therapists, and social workers. Physical therapists teach people how to perform exercises prescribed by doctors, and help them carry out the ones they cannot do alone or without special equipment. Physical therapists also explain the use of various methods to relieve pain, such as heat and cold treatments. Occupational therapists show people with arthritis how to perform tasks associated with their jobs or with daily activities. They suggest ways of improving efficiency by redesigning work areas, and demonstrate how certain devices and aids can help make routine activities such as bathing and dressing easier to do. They can make splints to rest joints and help prevent deformity. Social workers guide people to sources of help for environmental, financial, or emotional difficulties related to arthritis. Also, some counties have nursing services through which trained nurses (or, sometimes, physical therapists) visit the homes of people with serious arthritis or other diseases. These nurses or therapists monitor the person's condition, help perform or explain the prescribed treatment program, and note the person's response to this program.

No matter how many people are involved in the medical team that cares for someone with arthritis, the most important member is the person with arthritis. If you are that person, you must be a full partner in the effort to keep your disease under control; otherwise, your treatment will not be as effective as it should be. As a team member, you have several responsibilities. First, you need to have a positive attitude by focusing on how much you can still do despite the arthritis, rather than on the limits created by the arthritis. A second responsibility is to be open and honest at all times with physicians and all other members of the treatment team. Only the person with arthritis really knows how he or she feels. The more information the physician has about you, and about the effects of your arthritis and its treatment, the better he or she can work with you to overcome the disease. For this reason, persons with arthritis must keep their doctors fully informed of all aspects of their physical and emotional health. This includes explaining all noticeable symptoms and describing what relieves or increases the symptoms. Your worries and concerns must also be brought out into the open, so that your physician can help you understand and cope with your condition.

Finally, although the doctor and perhaps other health specialists will design the treatment program that is best suited to you, you have the responsibility of following it. Only you can be sure to follow the exercises closely, to take medications as prescribed, to get enough rest, to protect your joints from added stress, and to report any setbacks or progress in your treatment. This responsiblity calls for a lot of patience, since the results sometimes show up only after weeks or months of following a treatment program. The responsibility also requires flexibility in adjusting to the unpredictable ups and downs of a chronic rheumatic disease. But once it becomes routine, full participation in the treatment program becomes second nature for many people.

CHAPTER TWO

Understanding Arthritis

An important first step toward adjusting to arthritis is learning as much as possible about it. People who understand their condition and the reasons behind their doctors' recommendations are more apt than others to adapt well to the necessary limitations. Such knowledge is especially important for people with chronic diseases. They learn why certain changes may occur and what to do about them. They learn how to attain the best health they can expect. By seeking information, they have chosen not to be passively controlled by their diseases, but to learn to manage their health actively. These people can share important observations with their health professionals, to the benefit of the entire treatment team, and most important, to themselves.

People who have been recently diagnosed as having arthritis are usually full of questions. They want to know how their bodies are affected and what the future holds for their health. What does a joint look like? How does it change because of arthritis? What caused the disease in the first place? Are there cures? What's the latest on research?

Not all of the answers to these questions have been found, but researchers are currently following many promising leads. Today, scientists are well on their way to pinpointing causes of some of the major forms of arthritis. They are also getting closer to finding drugs that will be able to stop the diseases in their tracks.

Knowledge of the rheumatic diseases today is a far cry from

what it was in the first half of this century. At the time the Arthritis Foundation was formed in 1948, medical scientists lacked a well-defined approach to the study of the rheumatic diseases, and had only a few good leads to follow. Much research was limited to describing the effects of the various kinds of arthritis. There were no investigations of the pattern of how each disease occurs in the population, and no experimental models for scientists to use in studying arthritis. Now, many useful drugs are available, and more are in the testing stages. Excellent animal models allow researchers to study certain kinds of arthritis in ways they cannot do in humans. Large-scale studies currently underway should explain more about who gets arthritis and what kind of arthritis they develop, and in some situations should help define the circumstances that are likely to trigger a form of arthritis.

Leading researchers agree that the most likely causes of many rheumatic diseases involve interactions between an inherited susceptibility to these diseases, infections that trigger the disease process, chronic inflammation, and an unbalanced immune system. Each of these areas is a field of major research activity. But what do these terms mean, and how do these factors combine to affect joints and other parts of the body?

JOINT STRUCTURE

Before exploring what happens in arthritis-related disorders, it is important to understand the tissues that are affected. In most rheumatic diseases, one or more joints are affected. A joint is any place in the body where two bones meet. The ends of the bones are covered by cartilage, which is a tough, elastic tissue that acts as a shock absorber and keeps the bones from rubbing against each other. The entire joint is enclosed in a capsule that is lined by an inner membrane known as the synovial membrane. The membrane forms a slippery fluid, the synovial fluid, which fills the small space around and between the two bones. The synovial fluid nourishes the cartilage (which has no blood vessels) and keeps the joint lubricated, making movement smooth and easy.

Just outside the joint are muscles, tendons, and ligaments. These structures provide support and help the bones move in the right directions. Tendons are strong, cordlike structures that attach muscles to bones. Ligaments are similar to tendons

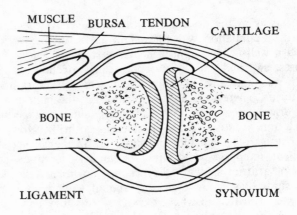

Joint anatomy

except that they connect the bones to each other. Fluid-filled sacs called bursae are spread among the muscles, bones, ligaments, and tendons, and help keep these structures moving smoothly against each other.

All of these tissues—the cartilage, muscles, ligaments, tendons, and synovial membranes—are made of different kinds of connective tissue. Connective tissue can be compared to the mortar that holds a brick building together. It is found throughout the body, and acts in varying capacities to form the body's support structures and keep the internal organs in place. Connective tissue also helps form the skin. Some rheumatic diseases (e.g., systemic lupus erythematosus, or lupus) affect many kinds of connective tissue in the body; others (e.g., osteoarthritis) are confined to only a few kinds of connective tissue.

INFLAMMATION

Many people with arthritis are familiar with the signs of inflammation—the heat, swelling, pain, redness, and loss of motion that occur in affected joints. Inflammation can occur anywhere in the body as a result of local tissue damage caused by events such as sports injuries, infections, animal or insect bites, and wounds. It is one of the ways in which the body protects itself from injury or the threat of disease. Inflammation is a normal process of protection and repair, and should subside once the damage has improved.

In many forms of arthritis, however, the inflammatory process goes out of control; it doesn't subside when it should, and leads to further tissue damage rather than tissue repair. Scientists don't know what event triggers and perpetuates the inflammation in most forms of arthritis, but most believe infections are partly to blame.

Until fairly recently, scientists did not understand the process of inflammation very well. Now, however, they are unraveling the sequence of events that occurs in this process, and finding it extremely intricate. Research on inflammation is one of the most exciting and promising fields of scientific endeavor today.

The inflammatory reaction begins with some sort of tissue irritation or damage (known as a "triggering" event). In response, many different kinds of white blood cells rush from the bloodstream into the area. They release enzymes and other active chemicals that affect the nearby cells and alter blood flow in the area.

Among the important chemicals released by the white blood cells are toxic (poisonous) substances made from molecular oxygen. They include superoxide radicals and hydrogen peroxide. Although these substances are valuable when the white blood cells use them to kill bacteria, such as in the event of infection, they can also harm nearby tissue cells.

Other active products released by the white blood cells include two related groups of chemicals known as prostaglandins and leukotrienes. Prostaglandins have a dual role in mediating inflammation; some kinds intensify the process and others slow it down. Leukotrienes, which were first recognized in 1979, are the most potent producers of inflammation yet known.

What do the prostaglandins and leukotrienes do? Some cause nearby cells to leak destructive enzymes and other substances into the inflamed area. They also increase the flow of fluids and white blood cells from tiny blood vessels into the area surrounding the inflammation. New white blood cells are then attracted to the inflamed area and release more prostaglandins and leukotrienes. The accumulation of these fluids and cells is what causes the swelling that accompanies an inflammation.

Prostaglandins and leukotrienes are produced by a complicated process. This begins with some triggering event that stimulates the membrane surrounding the white cell. A substance in the membrane, called arachidonic acid, then changes, in a series of chemical steps into twenty to thirty different compounds. These compounds include the different prostaglandins and leukotrienes, which are then released from the white cell.

Working out the complicated pathways by which prostaglandins and leukotrienes are produced and released has allowed researchers to search for agents that inhibit or interfere with this production. Several such agents are now being studied intensively for their effects on inflammatory cells in test tubes and in animals that have arthritis. Such studies have also partly shown that aspirin and the related nonsteroidal anti-inflammatory drugs help people with arthritis by interfering with prostaglandin production.

During inflammation, white blood cells also release a large number of digestive enzymes. Ordinarily, these enzymes are stored inside the white cells in sacs called lysosomes. Their primary job is to help these cells digest bacteria and remove compounds that form during the body's fight against invading infectious agents such as viruses or fungi. Sometimes, however, these enzymes spill out of the white cells into surrounding tissues, where they digest cartilage, bone, ligaments, muscles, and other tissues. The enzymes can be very destructive, and this is especially true of the enzyme called collagenase, which breaks down collagen, the main structural protein of connective tissue.

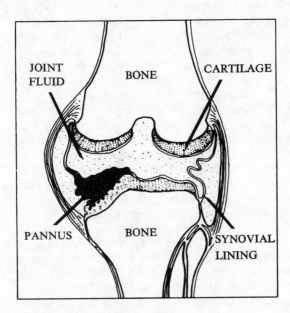

An inflamed joint

All of the foregoing substances released by white blood cells —superoxides, hydrogen peroxide, prostaglandins, leukotrienes, and digestive enzymes—are present in the inflamed joint. Here they interact with each other and with other inflammatory chemicals. The presence of these substances attracts still more white blood cells into the inflamed area, thereby feeding the process. In the inflammatory rheumatic diseases, this process may become chronic, and may cause significant damage to the joint tissues. In rheumatoid arthritis, inflammatory cells and fluid that accumulate in the synovium of the joint may create a growth called a pannus, which is a tongue of thickened, inflamed synovium. Substances in this mass eat into and damage the nearby cartilage. Under this attack, the cartilage softens, weakens, and may ultimately be destroyed. The destruction of cartilage throws off an assortment of substances and debris, attracting more inflammatory cells to the area.

THE IMMUNE SYSTEM

The immune system has the function of protecting the body against infection. Its overall duty is to distinguish between the body's own normal substances and "foreign" substances or agents such as viruses, bacteria, cancer cells, or fungi—which are known as antigens—and to attack these foreign substances. In many forms of arthritis, especially rheumatoid arthritis, the lack of control of inflammation probably stems from a malfunctioning immune system. The immune system errs at some point and mistakenly attacks normal tissues as if they were antigens.

The immune system has a myriad of defenses against antigens. These defense actions—of which inflammation is one— are carried out by the cells that make up the system, which include more than one trillion specialized white blood cells known as lymphocytes. There are different kinds of lymphocytes, with different actions; some kinds step up the attack against antigens; others slow it down. Specifically, there are two major categories of lymphocytes: T lymphocytes and B lymphocytes. B lymphocytes produce antibodies that combine with specific antigens such as bacteria to inactivate them. T lymphocytes regulate the production of antibodies by B lymphocytes. Some T lymphocytes, helper cells, stimulate B lymphocytes to produce antibodies. Other T lymphocytes, suppressor cells, turn off

15

antibody production by B cells. A third class of T cells, cytotoxic cells, can destroy cells containing certain antigens. All of
these lymphocytes work together to mount a balanced response
when necessary and to turn it off when the potential threat is
no longer serious.

How does the immune system swing into action when an
antigen appears in the body? The first major response is that the
antigen is recognized as such by another special cell called a
macrophage. The macrophage presents the antigen, in turn, to
a helper T cell and subsequently to a B cell. Rapid production
of T and B cells ensues.

The antibodies that are formed by the B cells seek out and
lock onto antigens to form compounds known as immune complexes. These complexes, in turn, trigger the complement system, a group of proteins that circulate in the blood. Through a
series of reactions, the complement system promotes inflammation by causing white cells to leak out of the blood into a tissue
such as a joint. The system also causes immune complexes to
be digested by macrophages, which reside in the tissues and
contain enzymes capable of digesting such complexes. As a

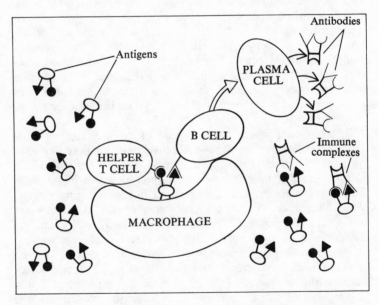

The formation of antibodies as part of the inflammatory response

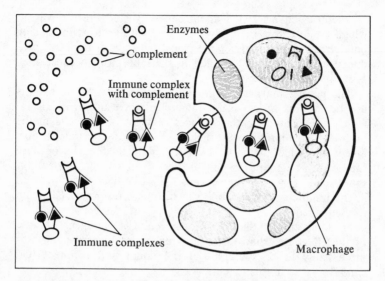

The ingestion of immune complexes as part of the inflammatory response

result of these different defense mechanisms, the threat posed by the antigen is usually removed. If everything functions properly, various control mechanisms then modify the immune response and the inflammation and eventually turn them off. These mechanisms include the actions of suppressor T cells and of prostaglandins that reduce inflammation. In some of the rheumatic diseases immune complexes continue to be formed and the production of antibodies is not turned off. Also in some diseases, especially lupus erythematosus, the mechanism for removing complexes is defective. Thus, the complexes continue to activate the complement, which in turn promotes an influx of white cells into the joint or other tissue, perpetuating the process of inflammation.

INHERITED TENDENCIES

Research has revealed that the tendency to get certain kinds of arthritis can be inherited. In other words, certain traits that predispose people to some of the rheumatic diseases can be passed in the genes from one generation to the next.

17

Scientists have learned about genes by studying the way in which they express themselves in the body, such as in causing hair or eye color. Some of the traits or "genetic markers" produced by genes can be studied in the laboratory because they occur in the form of proteins.

The genetic markers of greatest interest to arthritis experts are the proteins known as the human leukocyte antigens (HLA), which are located on the surfaces of most of the cells in the body. These markers were first discovered in the late 1960s. Scientists called them the human leukocyte antigens because they were first found on the surface of human leukocytes, another name for white blood cells. These antigens are involved in the immune system's ability to distinguish normal cells from foreign invaders.

Scientists first studied the human leukocyte antigens because of the effect they had on organ transplants. A transplant was more likely to be successful if the donor and recipient had similar or matching antigens.

Some years later, certain genetic markers were found to be associated with certain kinds of disease. These diseases included four major kinds of rheumatic disease: ankylosing spondylitis, rheumatoid arthritis, some forms of juvenile arthritis, and Reiter's syndrome (a form of arthritis that may develop as a complication of certain infections).

The first clue to a relationship between the human leukocyte antigens and rheumatic diseases came in 1973. Scientists found an overwhelming association of one HLA marker known as HLA-B27 with ankylosing spondylitis and Reiter's syndrome. This marker is found in eight percent of white people and two percent of black people, but in ninety-five percent of white people and fifty percent of American black people with ankylosing spondylitis. The HLA-B27 antigen is also found in a high proportion of the symptom-free relatives of these people. Although the presence of this marker conveys a susceptibiilty to ankylosing spondylitis, fewer than one in five HLA-B27 carriers actually develops the disease.

Genetic studies of children with certain kinds of juvenile arthritis have led to several discoveries. Thus, for example, several different diseases had for years been grouped together under the single name of juvenile rheumatoid arthritis. That this condition actually comprised different diseases had been suspected, but the differences were not fully understood until studies revealed associations of each of these diseases with different genetic markers. Researchers found, for example, that the presence of the HLA-B27 marker helped them identify an early form of what appears to be either ankylosing spondylitis or Reiter's syndrome in children who had been previously diagnosed as having juvenile rheumatoid arthritis.

Ankylosing spondylitis affects about two in one thousand white people. It was previously considered to be very rare in women. Today, as a result of studies of the HLA system, scientists know that ankylosing spondylitis may occur in a mild form in a larger number of people, and that women develop the disease far more often than doctors formerly thought.

Genetic studies have shown that more than sixty percent of adults with rheumatoid arthritis have a marker antigen called HLA-DR4. This marker is found in only twenty-seven percent of adults without rheumatoid arthritis; it occurs on the surface of B cells, the lymphocytes that produce antibodies, and is entirely different from the HLA-B27 marker.

Researchers hope that by studying the roles these genetic markers have in the body's normal functioning, they may find out what goes wrong in people who develop arthritis. This discovery would be a tremendous step toward understanding what causes the rheumatic diseases.

Someday, doctors may use such discoveries to identify people who are at risk for developing a particular kind of arthritis. A person's HLA markers can be identified through blood tests somewhat similar to tests done for blood typing. Although in theory, the identification of a certain disease-associated HLA marker might enable a person to avoid the disease, the current understanding of these markers is not good enough to warrant testing people to see which of the markers they have (if any), other than for research purposes.

Research on genetic markers and their influence in certain rheumatic diseases may eventually also lead to new approaches to the treatment of these diseases. For example, people with different genetic markers may respond differently to certain medications. People with rheumatoid arthritis who have inherited the HLA-DR4 marker do not improve as much with gold treatment as those who lack this marker, according to some studies. Perhaps doctors will be able to tailor drug treatment more closely to individual genetic traits and achieve better responses.

INFECTIOUS TRIGGERING AGENTS

Although some HLA markers are signposts of a person's susceptibility to certain rheumatic diseases, not everyone who inherits one of these markers actually develops the associated disease. Sometimes people who don't have any of the related genetic markers develop a rheumatic disease. Scientists are trying to find out why.

The idea is not new. For years, certain forms of arthritis were thought to be infectious diseases and many attempts were made to isolate bacteria as the cause of rheumatoid arthritis, but no infectious agents could be found. Infectious agents including bacteria, mycoplasma (an infectious agent similar to bacteria), bedsonia (another infectious agent resembling viruses), and viruses have been reported as being present in people with rheumatoid arthritis and other rheumatic diseases. So far, however, none of these reports has been confirmed.

Beyond this, recent research has revealed that several types of arthritis can occur as complications of infections. One example is the arthritis caused by Lyme disease, named for the Connecticut town where it was first recognized. The disease is transmitted by a tick bite, and usually begins with a small, red rash at the site of the bite. The rash typically spreads and is followed by vomiting, fever, headache, and neck stiffness. Later, some people develop severe joint inflammation, usually in the knees. The arthritis may subside after several weeks or months, or may recur and become chronic.

Only recently did scientists find that Lyme disease is caused by a spirochete, a type of bacterium. The spirochetes were found inside the ticks and in the blood and spinal fluid of some people who had the disease. In 1983, scientists devised a blood test that could reveal whether persons suspected of having Lyme disease had antibodies to the spirochete. If these antibodies are found, the diagnosis is confirmed, and treatment with antibiotics can begin promptly before damage to joints or other tissues becomes serious. The availability of this test is important because the spirochete itself is difficult to isolate from the blood.

Although these discoveries are important for people who live in areas where spirochete-carrying ticks are found, they also have exciting implications for other kinds of arthritis. They prove, for example, that chronic arthritis can result from an infection, and they permit at least this one form of arthritis to be monitored closely from the very beginning—even before the telltale signs of arthritis have developed. Thus, Lyme disease may provide researchers with subtle clues that will help them recognize very early the signs of a developing form of arthritis. Beyond this, the findings in Lyme disease also lend credence to the belief that other rheumatic diseases, such as rheumatoid arthritis, could result from infections that had occurred years earlier. Were this to be the case, it would explain the difficulty of isolating an infectious agent from persons with rheumatoid arthritis, for by the time the arthritis has developed, it may be too late to recover the agent.

Another rheumatic disease associated with infections is Reiter's syndrome. Many people with Reiter's syndrome develop it as a complication of infections of their bowels or genitourinary systems with certain bacteria such as shigella and yersinia. Several different kinds of these infections may trigger the syndrome, although scientists are not sure whether or how they actually cause it or lead to it.

Strong evidence indicates that infectious agents are related to the development of both Lyme arthritis and Reiter's syndrome. Another example of an infectious agent associated with an arthritic condition is the virus that causes hepatitis; after infection, some people develop arthritis either before or after they develop liver disease. The leads are much slimmer in linking rheumatoid arthritis to an infection, but research on the development of Lyme arthritis, Reiter's syndrome, and other kinds of infectious arthritis should provide better ideas of what to look for in rheumatoid arthritis. Perhaps more than one infectious agent, or several agents in a particular combination, is involved in this disease. The individual causative agent or combination may be different in different people.

IMMUNE-SYSTEM MALFUNCTIONS

A popular theory among arthritis experts is that some people's immune systems respond abnormally to infections, resulting in chronic inflammation. Since genetic markers in mice called H-2, resemble HLA, are known to control specific immune responses and because some immune diseases in mice are closely related to these H-2 genes, it is possible that a similar relationship exists in humans. For example, immunization of mice with collagen can produce a form of arthritis.

However, the disease only develops in mice that possess a certain H-2 gene that is required for a mouse to make antibodies to collagen. Somehow this gene controls the ability of the mouse to make a specific antibody.

What kinds of immune-system malfunctions occur in arthritis? Instead of effectively defending the body from disease, the immune system mistakenly seems to turn against the body and become part of the disease process.

In rheumatoid arthritis, systemic lupus, and some other rheumatic diseases, the removal of immune complexes may not proceed correctly. The continued presence of many immune complexes fuels inflammation. People with rheumatoid arthritis and lupus also have a strong capacity to overproduce certain antibodies. The antibodies are directed against parts of the person's own body cells rather than against invading antigens. Such antibodies are called autoantibodies and the diseases are termed autoimmune. The immune complexes formed by the combination of the autoantibodies with their antigens are largely responsible for the kidney damage that occurs in lupus.

Researchers know that in some ways the immune systems of people with some rheumatic diseases are hyperactive. At the same time, other functions of these people's immune systems are suppressed. This dichotomy has stimulated research into how the various kinds of immune cells interact with each other in these diseases. For example, scientists think that the suppressor T cells of some people with rheumatoid arthritis, lupus, or other diseases may be faulty or too scarce, and therefore cannot adequately control the production of antibodies by B cells.

In a few people with lupus, errors occur in the complement system which interacts with immune complexes to cause white cells to migrate into a joint or other organ. Some people are born lacking one of the proteins of the complement system. On the other hand, activation of a normal complement system can promote inflammation and contribute to kidney damage in other people with lupus.

Chronic inflammation may also result from an overproduction of those particular prostaglandins that promote inflammation. Indeed, this hypothesis is supported by the evidence that aspirin and anti-inflammatory drugs are also believed to block prostaglandin formation.

On the other hand, no one has proven that ankylosing spondylitis involves a faulty immune system. People with this form of spinal arthritis do not show many of the typical signs of immune-system abnormality that are found in rheumatoid arthritis and lupus. Nor are the effects of inflammation in ankylosing spondylitis the same as in other forms of arthritis. The inflammation proceeds at a much slower rate than in rheumatoid arthritis. Instead of destroying bone, the process results in excessive formation of new bone, causing the bones forming a joint to become fused.

Research into the function of the immune system in juvenile arthritis is similar in many ways to research in adult rheumatoid arthritis. Children who have had chronic, active disease for many years may have abnormal immune reactions. These reactions can be measured in the blood and the joint fluid; they are important in the development of the disease and probably sustain it. Children who appear to have fewer immune abnormalities respond better to treatment and their disease often disappears completely.

Researchers are trying to learn why some children develop certain autoantibodies and others do not. For example, children who have arthritis in only a few joints (pauciarticular juvenile rheumatoid arthritis) often develop eye disease that can lead to blindness. Such children often have an autoantibody in their blood that can react with the nuclei of human cells. This antibody is absent from children with other types of arthritis. Some other children with arthritis produce an antibody against T lymphocytes. The tendency to make these antibodies may be controlled by genes.

Although the cause and cure of many kinds of arthritis still elude scientists, exciting research results have provided solid leads in a wide variety of topics. People with arthritis can share the hope of experts that most forms of rheumatic disease will eventually yield to modern science. Until then, the progress already made against such disease since the 1950s has already rendered many forms of it controllable even if not curable.

CHAPTER THREE

Diagnosis

Discovering which kind of arthritis a person has is not always an easy task. Many forms of arthritis cause similar symptoms, especially in their early stages. Nor, with rare exceptions, do laboratory tests give absolute proof of a specific kind of arthritis. The most important parts of the diagnostic process are a careful medical history, including a full discussion of the current symptoms, and a physical examination. Laboratory tests are used primarily to add further support to the physician's diagnosis.

Some forms of arthritis can be diagnosed after only one or two visits with a physician. Others require several visits over a period of weeks or months, during which the pattern of the disease becomes clear. Some people need to spend time in a hospital while the diagnosis is being made and treatment is started. Occasionally, the doctor will make a tentative diagnosis, while waiting to see if later developments confirm that diagnosis.

HISTORY AND PHYSICAL EXAMINATION

The physician begins the search for a diagnosis with a detailed question-and-answer session pertaining to the person's symptoms. For people with symptoms associated with rheumatic diseases, examples of questions the doctor may ask are listed below:

- Where are the aches and pains?
- What makes them worse or better?
- Have any joints become warm and swollen?
- Which joints?
- At what time of day is the pain and stiffness most obvious?
- What past or recent injuries could have led to the joint inflammation?
- Have you had any fever? Chills? Unexplained weight loss?
- Are you more tired than usual?
- Do you have a skin rash? Bowel problems? Shortness of breath?
- What medications are you taking, including nonprescription drugs?

Many people find it helpful to bring a list of their symptoms and questions to the doctor so that they won't forget anything. This part of the diagnostic process is very important; it gives the doctor leads to the kinds of diseases that might be present, and helps the doctor decide which tests are needed and how to approach the physical examination.

During the physical examination, the doctor tries to determine the person's overall state of health and to zero in on the specific disease that may be present. This process involves paying close attention to the affected areas, such as the joints, muscles, and skin. The person may be asked to move certain joints and report if the movements cause pain, and if so where the pain is strongest. The doctor looks for the typical effects of each suspected disease, such as a particular rash found in one form of juvenile arthritis.

With this background information, the physician decides whether to order laboratory tests or X-rays. Sometimes, such tests are unnecessary because the proper diagnosis does not depend on them. In other situations, the physician needs a few tests to confirm a suspicion or further limit the possibilities for diagnosis.

Physicians use a wide range of tests to help diagnose different kinds of arthritis, but for any one person, the diagnosis will usually require only a few such tests. The following list explains the tests used most often.

BLOOD TESTS

Complete Blood Count

Counts of different types of blood cells are used in the diagnosis of many diseases. They are often done during the first office visit, and may be repeated during treatment to check on the person's progress. Red blood cells are evaluated using the hemoglobin test and the hematocrit. Hemoglobin is the protein in red cells that carries oxygen from the lungs to the tissues. The hematocrit measures the quantity of red cells present. The blood of persons with chronic inflammation due to arthritis often contains a low number of red blood cells (anemia).

The number of white blood cells may also be counted. A high white blood count may mean that an infection is present. A low count may be a side effect of drug treatment but is often present in untreated lupus erythematosus.

Less often, the blood components called platelets are counted. Because the platelets help the blood to clot, a low platelet count is a clue that there may be a bleeding problem. Some drugs used to treat arthritis, such as gold and penicillamine, can sometimes reduce the platelet count.

Erythrocyte Sedimentation Rate

This test, also called the ESR or sed rate, is a measurement of how fast the red blood cells fall, or sediment, to the bottom of a glass tube that is filled with whole blood and allowed to sit for an hour. People with inflammation due to arthritis or any other cause usually have higher sedimentation rates than normal. If they improve with treatment, the sedimentation rate usually drops.

Antibody Tests

There are several blood tests for abnormal antibodies that suggest the presence of certain forms of arthritis. One is called the rheumatoid factor (RF) test, or RA latex test. It measures whether a certain kind of abnormal antibody called rheumatoid factor is present in the blood, and if so, how much is present. Rheumatoid factor is an antibody against the gamma globulin fraction of the blood. Since gamma globulin itself represents antibody molecules, rheumatoid factor is an antibody against other antibodies. Most people with rheumatoid arthritis have large amounts of RF in their blood.

Another test for abnormal antibodies is called the antinuclear antibody (ANA) test. It detects a group of autoantibodies that are found in most people with lupus and scleroderma, and in a few people with rheumatoid arthritis. One of the antinuclear antibodies, called anti-DNA, is especially important in the diagnosis of lupus. This autoantibody reacts with DNA, the chemical material in the nucleus of a cell that makes up the genes. Other ANAs are helpful in the diagnosis of certain other rheumatic diseases such as scleroderma, polymyositis, and Sjogren's Syndrome.

Complement Test

The complement system consists of a group of blood substances (as described in Chapter 2) that help antibodies to fight disease-causing agents that have entered the body by promoting inflammation. The complement test measures the amount of complement in the blood; people with active lupus often have lower than normal amounts of complement, especially if the kidneys are affected.

Muscle Enzyme Tests

In some rheumatic diseases, the muscles are damaged and release certain enzymes that they normally contain into the blood. Various tests can be used to measure the amount of these enzymes in the blood, helping the physician to judge whether one of these diseases is present, and how seriously it has damaged the muscles. Later on, muscle enzyme tests help show whether drug therapy has been effective. Some of these enzymes can also be elevated in the blood as a result of liver disease and other causes.

Creatinine Test

In certain kinds of arthritis, the kidneys may be affected. If the doctor suspects that they have, a test may be done to determine the amount of a normal waste product called creatinine in the blood. A high level may mean that the kidneys are not working well enough to remove wastes from the body.

Uric Acid Test

Blood can be tested for the amount of uric acid (a waste product of the urine) it contains. People with gout have elevated levels of uric acid, a condition called hyperuricemia. However, it is common to have hyperuricemia without ever getting gout.

URINE TESTS

Some tests of the urine may be done in people suspected of having arthritis. Urinalysis consists of a series of tests done to determine the contents of the urine. The tests show whether the urine contains red blood cells, protein, or a variety of abnormal substances, none of which is normally present. The detection of these substances may indicate kidney damage in certain rheumatic diseases, such as lupus, as well as the side effects of some drugs used in treating arthritis.

Occasionally, more detailed information is needed, and the physician will order twenty-four-hour urine tests. In these, all of the urine passed during a twenty-four-hour period is collected and analyzed for the amount of various different substances. This test shows how fast these substances are being passed into the urine, and may give more accurate results than are given by a one-time urinalysis.

TESTS OF THE JOINT FLUID

Sometimes it is helpful for the doctor to remove and examine some fluid from an inflamed joint. This procedure, called joint aspiration, is done by inserting a needle into the joint and withdrawing the fluid. Examination of the fluid may show whether the inflammation is caused by an infection or by the presence of crystals, such as the uric acid crystals that form in the joints in gout and calcium pyrophosphate crystals in pseudogout. If an infection is found, the specific bacteria that are causing it can be identified and the most effective antibiotic can be prescribed. If crystals are found, appropriate drug therapy can begin.

BIOPSIES

The word biopsy means the removal and examination of some tissue for use in making a diagnosis. Several different kinds of biopsies may be used to diagnose a rheumatic condition, some of which can be done in the doctor's office. One is a muscle biopsy, in which a bit of muscle is removed and examined with a microscope for signs of damage to the muscle fibers. Such

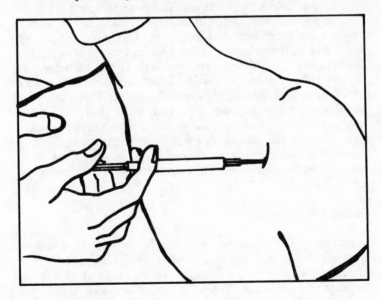

Joint aspiration

29

damage may mean the presence of a rheumatic disease called polymyositis.

Biopsies may also be performed on the skin, which may be affected in several forms of arthritis including lupus, sclero-derma, or psoriatic arthritis, or in a group of blood vessel diseases called the arteritides, which are sometimes associated with arthritis. If the doctor suspects a certain kind of rheumatic disease known as temporal arteritis, a tiny sample of tissue from one of the arteries near the temples is removed and examined for signs of damage.

A biopsy of a kidney may be done if the physician thinks the kidneys are damaged, as can occur in lupus. This procedure is done by passing a needle through the back into the kidney and withdrawing a bit of tissue for examination. In rare circumstances, a biopsy of the joint lining, or synovium, may be done. For this test, a needle is inserted into the joint and a small piece of tissue is removed.

ARTHROSCOPY

Arthroscopy is a relatively new kind of procedure for directly viewing the insides of the joints. The procedure is done in an operating room, where an orthopedic surgeon inserts an arthroscope, a small periscope-like instrument (often only one-eighth of an inch in diameter), into the joint and moves it around to examine the joint tissues, and particularly the cartilage, for damage. The person on whom arthroscopy is done may be under general anesthesia (completely put to sleep) or local anesthesia (in which a part of the body is numbed). If a treatable condition is found, the surgeon can often perform surgery right through the arthroscope using tiny instruments. Instruments may also be inserted through another hole in the joint. See Chapter Seven for more information on arthroscopic surgery.

X-RAYS

Although X-rays may occasionally be valuable in making a diagnosis when the symptoms of a rheumatic disease first appear, they are not very useful in the diagnosis of most kinds of arthritis unless the disease is fairly advanced. Early on, damage to the bones and cartilage is not extensive enough to

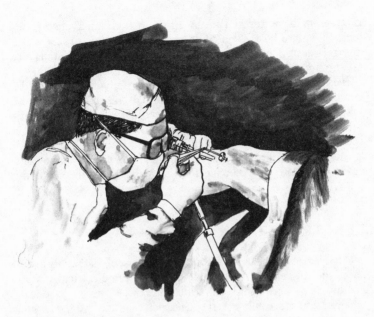

Arthroscopic examination

show up on X-rays. Often, the X-rays give confusing results: people with no symptoms may have abnormal X-rays and those with much pain can have normal ones. This situation is particularly true for people with back pain. X-rays taken early in the course of arthritis, however, are useful for comparison with later ones taken to see if the disease has progressed.

In some forms of arthritis, X-rays taken after the disease has been present for a long time may help in monitoring its progress. This type of evaluation is frequently done in people who have had rheumatoid arthritis for many years. Doctors also use X-rays to determine how well certain treatment programs are controlling bone damage and which people may need joint surgery. Diagnostically, X-rays are especially useful for identifying ankylosing spondylitis, for finding the bone growths called osteophytes which often develop in people with osteoarthritis, and for finding the crystals that cause the disease sometimes called pseudogout, but more correctly termed calcium pyrophosphate dihydrate crystal deposition disease, or CPPD disease.

Sometimes a special kind of X-ray procedure called a

myelogram is performed in an effort to find spinal disc problems that may be the cause of back pain. In this procedure, a dye is injected into the spinal canal, after which X-rays are taken and studied to see whether bulging discs are pressing on nerves and causing pain. Recently, a new X-ray technique called computerized tomography has permitted this diagnosis to be made in some people without the need for a myelogram. Another important X-ray method is arthrography, in which a special dye that coats cartilage is injected into the joint before an X-ray is taken. The physician can then visualize the joint cavity and note any damage to the cartilage surface or to the synovial lining.

ELECTROMYOGRAM

An electromyogram (EMG) is often used to diagnose diseases that affect the muscles. It measures the electrical pattern of muscles. The EMG can often help the physician decide whether muscle weakness results from rheumatic disease such as polymyositis (inflammation of the muscles), or a nerve disease instead. It is similar to an electrocardiogram (ECG or EKG), which measures the electrical pattern of the nerves and muscles in the heart. The nerves themselves can be tested by measuring the speed at which electrical impulses are carried along them. This measurement is known as the nerve conduction time. The conduction time is normal in polymyositis but prolonged if nerve damage is present.

Although the major portion of this chapter describes laboratory tests and other procedures for diagnosing the rheumatic diseases, it is important to remember that each person will probably need only a very few and perhaps none of these tests and procedures. Some tests are seldom used; others provide results that may not affect the treatment plan one way or another. The physician is in the best position to decide which ones need to be done and when, depending on the individual's condition as determined through the medical history and physical examination.

CHAPTER FOUR

Rest, Exercise, and Joint Protection

Although many people think that nothing can be done for arthritis, the truth is that most of those who follow a prescribed treatment program from early in the course of their disease will do well and can live full lives. Once the diagnosis of a certain kind of arthritis has been made, the physician works with the person to plan a full treatment program tailored to that person's specific disease and needs. The treatment is aimed at reducing pain and inflammation (if present); maintaining or increasing motion and strength; allowing the person to function as fully as possible without help; and preventing serious joint damage.

The results don't come easily or quickly, but if all aspects of the program are followed closely, they usually do come with time. Although the physician and other members of the health care team are responsible for planning the treatment program and advising about how to carry it out, its success depends on the individual for whom it is designed, who must accept the responsibility to follow the plan every day. Some people have trouble making this daily effort, but those who work at it often find that the changes become part of their daily routine and interfere little with their lives.

Although each treatment program differs according to each person's needs and state of health, the most comprehensive programs include pain control methods, therapeutic exercise, means to correct the posture, resting of the joints and the whole body, medication, and the use of devices and aids to help protect the joints. Occasionally, surgery may be necessary to repair badly damaged joints.

Not everyone with arthritis needs all of these aspects of treatment to manage his or her disease. The correct program for each individual depends on that individual's type of arthritis, its severity, and the general health and daily activities of the individual. For example, someone with osteoarthritis in one joint may not need such a complete program, whereas someone who has had serious rheumatoid arthritis for many years would require a full program.

This chapter focuses on the general concepts of rest, exercise, posture, and joint protection. The following chapters explain the uses of medications, pain control methods, and surgery for arthritis.

REST

A balanced mixture of rest and exercise is important for anyone with arthritis. This balance varies according to the severity of the symptoms and how easily the person tires. Doctors usually advise more rest and less exercise during flare-ups of the disease and greater exercise during its improved stages. Rest helps to control inflammation, and when balanced with exercise, helps in maintaining alertness and activity. Too much rest, however, may lead to increased fatigue and start a vicious cycle in which the person requires more rest, which creates more fatigue and so on. Such a cycle can become difficult to break and may result in stiff joints and withdrawal from activity.

On the other hand, because too much exercise may increase inflammation and damage the joints, the right balance between rest and exercise is important for the best control of arthritis. Doctors and therapists help each person to find that right balance. They may recommend scheduling short rest periods during the day, especially around lunchtime. People with arthritis must also be sure that they get enough sleep at night.

Relaxation is an important part of rest because it helps to reduce tension in the muscles and relieve pain. Some people can relax easily; others need to learn and practice specific techniques before they truly relax their bodies. Several useful methods are available for relaxation training, and different people may find they prefer certain of these over others. As long as the training leads to relaxation, the method chosen does not matter. Popular methods include progressive muscle relaxation and biofeedback.

Some relaxation techniques are similar to meditation. The person finds a comfortable position in a quiet environment and tries to empty his or her mind of all distracting thoughts, concentrating on breathing or pleasant feelings. Other relaxation methods involve alternately tensing and relaxing the various muscle groups throughout the body. This helps in feeling the difference between tense muscles and relaxed ones. Hatha yoga, transcendental meditation, hypnotic relaxation, autogenic training (self-hypnosis), Zen, and relaxation response are among these methods of relaxation through meditation.

Many persons with arthritis may also find it helpful to use a record or cassette specifically designed to assist them in meditation/relaxation technique.

Planning Ahead to Reduce Fatigue

Besides being alleviated by getting enough rest, fatigue can be reduced by carefully planning daily schedules. You can limit the amount of effort you need to keep up with your activities by thinking ahead, combining related tasks and errands, pacing yourself, and getting help from family members, friends, and co-workers. This planning calls for some flexibility, since the person with arthritis doesn't always know how tired or energetic he or she will be at certain times.

Here are several tips for scheduling daily activities. First, set definite priorities for your activities at home, at work, and during leisure time. Making a list of these activities can help you decide which are the most important, which can be modified to be less tiring, and which can be eliminated. For example, some housework chores can be cut back, spread out over several days, or shared with another member of your household. Tasks requiring much physical labor, such as reorganizing a large stockroom, can be done a little at a time. Different activities planned for the same day should be alternated between those that can be done while sitting and those that require standing or walking.

Rearrange your storage systems at home and work so that tools and gadgets for related tasks are within close reach, and the steps required to complete different tasks are reduced to the bare minimum. You can, for example, organize an area in the kitchen for preparing food while sitting by placing the tools needed for certain kinds of cooking (baking, for example) within easy reach of your seat. In an office, set up your work tables, desks, and storage areas so that getting the items you use most often does not require much reaching, walking, or bending. Wheeled tables and carts help reduce effort in many settings, such as home workshops, kitchens, game rooms, and repair shops. Occupational therapists can assist you in making all of these kinds of adjustments.

EXERCISE

Regular exercise is an important part of an arthritis treatment program. Here, exercise does not mean the kind pursued by an active, athletic person, such as vigorous sports or strenuous training sessions. Rather, it entails a planned program for building and keeping muscle strength, reducing fatigue, stabilizing and supporting the joints, and increasing or maintaining mobility. Strong muscles and ligaments help keep the joints in place and reduce unnecessary stress on them. Exercise also helps to keep the bones strong, and may nourish the joint cartilage by increasing its supply of synovial fluid.

When properly performed, exercises can help prevent or improve many joint deformities. They also help to distract attention from pain and everyday problems, and provide a sense of accomplishment as improvement occurs.

The plan of exercise differs from one person with arthritis to the next. The recommended program depends on the kind and severity of the arthritis, the person's physical condition, and which joints are involved. Because these factors vary widely, specific exercises or plans are not described here. Rather, our discussion will focus on the kinds of exercises that may be prescribed, and on general suggestions for starting and staying with an exericse program.

The exercises for persons with rheumatic disease can be categorized in several different ways. One way is to group them according to the desired results. Thus, there are exercises for improving a person's range-of-motion (stretching), muscle-strengthening exercises, and endurance exercises.

The phrase "range of motion" refers to all of the normal movements that a joint can make in different directions. Arthritis sometimes causes a reduction in the range of motion of

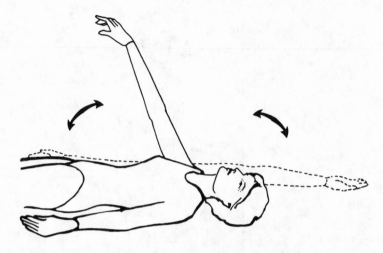

An example of a range-of-motion exercise: Lie on your back; raise one arm over your head, keeping your elbow straight; bring your arm close to your ear; return your arm slowly to your side. Repeat this exercise with your other arm; repeat, alternating arms.

the joints it affects. Unless stretching exercises are begun early enough, permanent joint deformity may result. The joint may get stuck in the bent position, in which case the person is said to have a "flexion contracture." Range-of-motion exercises are designed to prevent such contractures; they consist of gentle movements to the limits of each joint's motion. Gradually, these stretching exercises improve flexibility.

Strengthening exercises build up strength in muscles, ligaments, and tendons, the tissues that support the joints. Doctors and physical therapists often recommend isometric, or muscle-tightening, exercises to build strength. These exercises involve no movement of the joints, and therefore improve strength without adding stress to the joints. An example of isometric exercise is pushing against a wall to improve arm muscles.

Endurance or aerobic exercises are good for improving overall fitness. They complement range-of-motion and strengthening exercises. Examples of endurance exercises are walking, swimming, and bicycling. These activities build up heart and lung strength, and when fit into a balanced routine that includes enough rest, they help reduce chronic fatigue and maintain physical fitness.

37

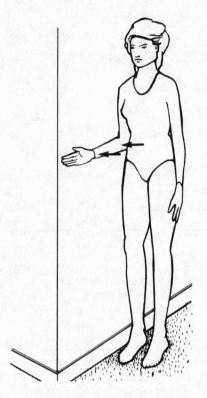

An example of an isometric exercise: Stand beside a wall with your arm, elbow, entire forearm and back of your hand against the wall; your elbow should be bent like an "L"; push your entire forearm (elbow, wrist, and hand) against the wall as if you are trying to push the wall away. Make sure you stand up straight and that you do NOT lean into the wall; hold for a slow count of five; release. Repeat five times with one arm, then five times with the other arm. You can also do this exercise by sitting in a chair and pushing against the side of the arm of the chair.

Exercises may also be categorized as either active or passive. All of the exercises described above are considered active; that is, the person moves his or her own body without the physical help of another person. Passive exercises are those in which a helper, such as a physical therapist or family member, moves the person's body for him. For example, while the person is lying down, the helper may lift his or her leg and move the hip through its range of motion. These exercises maintain range of motion during a period of active disease when a person cannot carry through the full range without assistance.

Exercise Guidelines

Several guidelines can help you get the most out of an exercise program.

Getting Started

The best way to begin is slowly and gently. You should try to increase the amount of exercise a little each day. Many people put off starting an exercise program, waiting until they feel better. Perhaps they would be more eager to begin exercising if they realized that regular use will improve their joints and muscles and help them feel better sooner than if they kept waiting.

Frequency

Generally, you should perform exercises twice or more each day. During each period, every exericse should be repeated several times, starting with a few times and gradually working up to many repetitions. People who have problems with fatigue should allow themselves several short exercise periods during the day rather than one long period.

Increasing Exercise

The goal of an exercise program is to improve joint and muscle function gradually. Exercises performed too vigorously or too often may increase the pain from and damage to diseased joints. It is important to maintain the right balance between too little exercise and too much.

Discomfort

Although some discomfort and minor pain may occur during exercises, strong or long-lasting pain means the exercises are being overdone. A general rule is that if increased pain lasts for more than about two hours after the end of an exercise period, you should inform your physician or therapist. The exercises may then be modified.

Assistance

At first, a helper may be needed to help the person with arthritis to be able to do some of the prescribed exercises. The helper should not force a joint through any motion that the person cannot do alone, but should rather assist only those motions that the person already can do, but which may be difficult. The person with arthritis should try to do as many exercises without help as possible. For special assistance, some people need to make a number of regular visits with a physical therapist.

When Joints Are Inflamed

When the joints are very painful and inflamed, exercise must be done gently, with a minimum of motion of the involved joints. The emphasis should be on isometric and range-of-motion exercises. A helper may be needed at such times.

When Inflammation Has Gone Down

When the joints are not too swollen or painful, the exercise program will generally focus on building strength in muscles, and on increasing or retaining motion so that normal activities can be carried out.

For Mild Arthritis

People who have a mild degree of arthritis may have an exercise program designed to strengthen their muscles, increase the movement of their joints, and improve their overall body condition. Your doctor or therapist can advise which sports are safe and which cause too much jarring or too many sudden, jerky movements.

POSTURE

Regular exercise goes hand in hand with correct posture. If you have poor posture, your exercise program won't work as well as it could. People with arthritis have a natural tendency to find a comfortable position for each painful joint, and to keep the joints in that position for long periods. Usually, these positions are ones in which the joints are bent to some degree. They may lead to the flexion contractures described earlier, in which joints become permanently "locked." To help prevent these contractures, regular exercises must be supplemented with good posture.

Correct posture can be achieved by following a few basic guidelines. In any position, you should strive to keep the back as straight as possible, so as to avoid putting too much stress on any group of muscles or joints. When standing, you should hold your head up, pull in your stomach, and keep your knees and hips straight and not cocked to one side. When you are walking, your arms should swing freely at your sides and your body weight should shift only slightly from side to side.

Keeping good posture when seated helps reduce fatigue and pain. The best position is one in which you sit up straight without slumping, with your head held up and your feet flat on the floor. If you must sit for long periods, stretch occasionally and move around to keep from getting too stiff. Use straight-backed chairs, preferably ones with arms, whenever possible.

When sitting at a desk or table, make sure that your arms and hands can reach the level of the workspace easily. Using a slanted table such as those used for drafting will help you avoid slumping while working.

People with arthritis should avoid sitting for long periods on the edges of beds or on soft chairs or couches. Lack of enough back support while seated encourages poor posture.

Good posture is just as important to maintain when lying down. Many doctors encourage people with arthritis to use firm mattresses and to put plywood boards between their inner springs and mattresses. Some people need to use sleeping and resting aids such as specially shaped pillows or footboards to maintain a proper posture while in bed. Doctors and physical or occupational therapists can explain how to use these aids.

Using the proper shoes also helps you maintain good posture. Low or flat heels put less stress on the lower back, legs, and hips than do high heels. They help people stand correctly and walk with ease. Also, comfortable shoes that are made of strong material provide more support to the feet and are less tiring to the legs than softer shoes. Some people with arthritis affecting their feet are helped by specially designed shoe inserts.

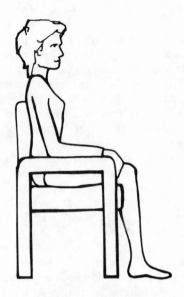

Correct sitting posture: Head and back are straight and in line with each other; buttocks are in contact with the back of the chair, and feet are placed firmly on the floor.

Physicians and podiatrists can explain the use of such inserts and recommend them if necessary. People with arthritis in the joints at the balls of the feet can obtain relief from a metatarsal bar, which is a triangular piece of leather added to the sole of the shoe in the forward part of the instep.

JOINT PROTECTION

Some people with arthritis have difficulty with routine activities such as bathing, cleaning, dressing, and so forth. Various simple devices are available that can be helpful in carrying out these and other tasks. These aids allow people to care for themselves and protect injured joints from added stress. Some examples of devices for use at home are grab bars for getting in and out of bathtubs or up from toilets, eating utensils with large handles, aids to help zip and unzip clothing, clothing made with easy-to-use fastenings, combs with extra long handles, and special doorknobs with flat levers that can be opened by push-

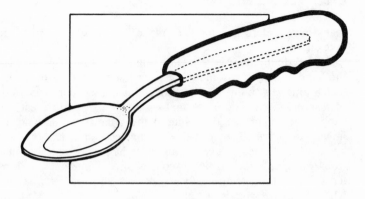

A spoon with a built-up handle is easier to grasp.

ing with the palm or elbow. Similar devices are made for use in many job settings. (For more information, the Arthritis Foundation publishes a "Self-Help Manual for Patients with Arthritis" which describes such devices and lists where to get them. See Chapter 26 for the address.)

Other Means of Protecting the Joints

Many other means are available to protect the joints from further damage and from becoming too stiff. For example, aids such as walkers, canes, and crutches help protect joints such as the hips, knees, ankles, and feet that must bear much of the body's weight by distributing this weight over a number of joints.

Doctors and therapists recommend the use of splints for some people to help rest and protect damaged joints, especially ones that are severely inflamed and developing deformities. The splints are used at night or during daytime rest breaks to hold the joints in the correct positions and to keep the muscles and ligaments around the joints limber. They help prevent contractures from developing and remind the wearer not to overuse specific joints. They are usually removed for exercise periods.

Many splints are custom-made. Several different kinds of plastics are used to make them, and plaster of paris is sometimes used to form a close fit between the splint and the affected joint. Many splints are padded with foam rubber, and many have Velcro fastenings to make them easy to put on and take off.

Three commonly used kinds of splints are a resting splint for the hand and wrist, a functional (working) splint for the wrist, and a long leg splint. The resting splint is used during periods of rest and sleep. The functional wrist splint is used to rest and support an inflamed wrist while at the same time allowing the fingers to move. The long leg splint rests and supports the knee while the leg is kept straight. It helps prevent the knee from becoming locked in a contracture. Sometimes a long leg splint is used temporarily to support and protect the knee while the wearer stands or walks.

Occasionally, splints may need to be replaced because: inflammation has increased or decreased the size of the joint, the joint's range of motion has changed, or the doctor decides that the soft tissues around the joint are ready to be stretched a little further. People using splints should tell their doctors or therapists of any discomfort they cause; these professionals may then

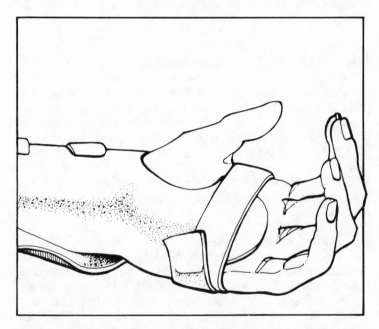

This splint helps rest and support an inflamed wrist, yet allows the fingers complete mobility.

alter or replace them. Such alterations should not be done by the user because an improper fit may actually cause more harm to the joint than if no splint were used.

Guidelines for Joint Protection

In addition to using resting splints, walking aids, and self-help devices as needed, people with arthritis can learn to protect their joints in other ways during daily activities. There are a few guidelines to help in learning these techniques:

- Large joints should be used whenever possible in place of small ones. For example, you should use a whole

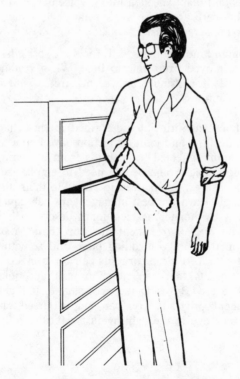

Using the hip or whole arm instead of one hand to shut doors will protect the small joints of the hand.

arm or hip rather than one hand to push doors open or to close cupboard doors.

- When lifting or pushing, spread the load out to as many joints as possible. For example, pick up a book with both arms instead of one.

- Joints should be used in their most natural positions; they should not be bent or twisted awkwardly, if possible. For example, when you're getting up out of chairs, don't twist your hips and back, but try to push yourself straight out of the chair with both arms.

- Examine all tasks for possible shortcuts and easier ways of getting them done. For example, a gardener should avoid repeated trips to the tool shed by loading all of the items and plants needed into a wheelbarrow to take out to the work area. Use the special devices described earlier to make tasks easier.

- Joints should not remain still for long periods, and should be moved from time to time. When reading for long periods, for instance, move and stretch your joints to prevent stiffness.

The guidelines and principles described in this chapter for rest, exercise, posture, and joint protection have important roles in preventing joints affected by arthritis from becoming badly damaged or deformed. Some people need to emphasize only a few of these measures; others need to attend to them all. Physicians help people learn the best management techniques on an individual basis. Although the techniques described here form only part of an overall treatment program that also includes medications, methods of controlling pain, and sometimes surgery, close attention to these concepts can often make a difference between joints that can function well and joints that become hard to use. By using the necessary techniques in the overall treatment program, you can help yourself and your doctors gain the edge in the fight against arthritis.

CHAPTER FIVE

Medication

Taking medication is a vital part of the treatment for most types of arthritis. When used as prescribed, drugs usually help the person with arthritis gain control over the effects of the disease. When used incorrectly, however, they can be dangerous to your health. For these reasons, people taking medicine need to understand several general concepts about drug therapy. Remember, medicine alone won't provide the best control of arthritis: it is only one part of a comprehensive treatment program.

There is no simple formula that doctors follow in deciding which medication to give to which person with arthritis. Many people may not know that the same drug can act differently in different people and that physicians have to prescribe drug treatments on an individual basis. What works well for one person may do no good for another. Moreover, even people with the same form of arthritis may be affected in very different ways by a drug, and their medicine may therefore be given with different goals in mind.

The choice of which arthritis medication to use depends on many factors. The doctor considers the kind of arthritis that is to be treated, how severe the disease is, the amount of pain, his or her prior experience in prescribing the appropriate drugs, the other drugs the person is taking, how well the person is likely to follow a suggested medicine schedule, and the person's overall health and age. Add to this list the fact that doctors have no good way of predicting how well a person's body will respond to a certain drug, and the selection becomes even more difficult. Sometimes, after a person has taken a medication for a while, the drug may stop working for no apparent reason, or may begin to cause unpleasant side effects such as nausea, a skin rash, or ringing in the ears. If this happens, the doctor must try to find a different drug for that person. Sometimes a person must keep trying several medicines over a period of years in an attempt to control his or her arthritis as much as possible. Although this searching process may be frustrating, the results are usually worth the effort and patience in the long run.

All drugs occasionally cause side effects, particularly when they are taken over a long period. Arthritis drugs are no exception. Each physician is aware of the side effects each of these drugs may cause, and takes them into account when choosing a drug to prescribe. The potential risks of a drug's side effects are weighed against its potential benefits in fighting the disease. This chapter will list major side effects of the arthritis drugs, but it is important to remember that a particular drug's side effects usually occur rarely, and that not all of the side effects develop in a single person. Further information about side effects is available through physicians, pharmacists, and local chapters of the Arthritis Foundation. The Arthritis Foundation publishes a series of Medication Briefs, each of which describes one of the commonly used drugs in the treatment of arthritis.

New drugs are continuously being developed for use in treating arthritis. Because they are first used experimentally, very few physcans are able to prescribe them for the people under their care. Many are strong and can have very serious side effects, and so cannot be used widely until they have been extensively tested.

Because the experimental tests on a new drug are done on a relatively small number of people with arthritis (five- to ten thousand), many rare side effects—some of which can be serious—do not become known until after the drug has been taken by 100,000 or even 1 million people. New drugs are often introduced with a great deal of publicity, some of it sensational. In general, it is not a good idea for people to try each new drug that comes on the market unless their physicians decide they are not getting beneficial effects from the medicine they are already taking. Rather, they should usually stay on the same medication programs until a new drug has had extensive use.

The person with arthritis can play an important role in ensuring that he or she receives the most benefit from a particular medicine. In order to do this you need to learn about your medications—their names, why they are important to take in the way the doctor directs, how to take them, how long to expect to keep taking them before they may begin to affect the arthritis, what their side effects may be, and what to do if side effects occur. It is also important to learn whether a drug prescribed for treating arthritis may interact with another drug you may be taking for a different condition.

People with arthritis must also work closely with their physicians in deciding whether their medications have improved their health. This responsibility includes taking special care to report all changes in your health, whether good or bad, and following the doctor's instructions exactly. The physician must also know if you have not taken your medication as directed for whatever reason—the bottle was lost, you forgot, and so forth. This honesty and cooperation keeps the doctor from drawing the wrong conclusions about the drug's effectiveness or about how your body tolerates the drug.

ARTHRITIS DRUGS

What drugs are used for arthritis? They range from the most familiar of medications, aspirin, to powerful drugs that may cause serious side effects. They fall into four general categories: aspirin and similar-acting medications, which are called the nonsteroidal anti-inflammatory drugs (NSAID); steroid drugs; slow-acting (or disease-modifying) drugs; and cytotoxic medications. Many doctors first try large doses of aspirin or NSAIDs. If these medications are not effective, they must consider selecting stronger ones, attempting to find the least potent medication that controls the pain and inflammation for a particular person. For people with severe forms of arthritis, physicians may have to try drugs that suppress the immune system. These drugs are very powerful and carry a substantial risk of serious side effects.

Aspirin

Aspirin is a time-honored medicine that is still one of the best choices for most people with many types of arthritis. The effects and importance of aspirin, however, are not well understood by most people. Because it is so common, can be bought without a prescription, and is used for everyday aches and pains, many people think that aspirin is too simple to use for painful rheumatic diseases. Some even wonder if their doctors are serious when they tell them to take aspirin for these diseases.

In fact, when taken in proper amounts, aspirin is an excellent drug for many kinds of arthritis. It reduces pain and inflammation and is one of the safest drugs on the market. The pain-relieving effect of aspirin works at lower doses (usually two tablets every four hours); however, a high level of aspirin is needed in the blood for the control of inflammation. At these high levels, aspirin blocks the production of the prostaglandins that help trigger and perpetuate inflammation. The aspirin level in the body must remain high for some time before the drug can produce its full benefit. When the proper level is achieved, generally in a few days, the person must usually keep taking aspirin at the same doses—even when he or she feels better. If this is not done, the symptoms may return.

Possible Side Effects

Some people who take high doses of aspirin day after day may experience side effects of nausea, indigestion, and vomiting. These side effects may sometimes be avoided by taking the drug with food or milk, or by crushing the aspirin tablets and putting the powder into yogurt or a large glass of water or milk. Special forms of aspirin are available that help some people avoid stomach upset. These include aspirin in liquid form, coated aspirin tablets, and time-released aspirin preparations.

Additional side effects resulting from high doses of aspirin are buzzing or ringing in the ears, dizziness, a slight loss of hearing, or changes in vision. These side effects will go away if the dosage is lowered or if the use of aspirin is stopped altogether.

A few people develop allergy-like symptoms of hay fever, asthma, hives, or a rash after taking aspirin. These symptoms can be serious. If you should experience any of them, stop taking aspirin and call your doctor right away.

Aspirin Brands

Many different brands of aspirin are available, and not all are equivalent. Besides the buffered, coated, and liquid forms, some brands contain ingredients other than aspirin. Such additions are not needed to help relieve the symptoms of arthritis, and usually make the product cost more than plain aspirin. Different brands also may contain different amounts of aspirin in each tablet. Unless the doctor suggests a certain kind of aspirin (e.g., buffered, liquid, or time-released), one brand is as good as another. The important point is to get the proper amount (a certain number of grains or milligrams). Often, unadvertised "house brands" are the cheapest, and give the same results as the more expensive brands.

The over-the-counter group of drugs called "aspirin substitutes" usually contain acetaminophen, which reduces pain but has no effect on inflammation. Thus, they are not as effective as aspirin for most forms of arthritis. People who are advised by their physician to take aspirin should ask the physician before trying one of the aspirin substitutes.

Nonsteroidal Anti-Inflammatory Drugs

Together with aspirin, the most commonly used category of drugs for arthritis are the nonsteroidal anti-inflammatory drugs (NSAIDs). The NSAIDs were given this name because they reduce inflammation like the cortisone (steroid) drugs do, but have important differences from the steroids and work in different ways. Technically, aspirin belongs to the NSAID group, but is usually considered apart from the other members. In this discussion, "NSAIDs" will refer to the drugs in this group other than aspirin.

The NSAIDs have about the same ability as aspirin to reduce pain and inflammation, and work in the same way—by blocking the formation of prostaglandins. There are some important differences between NSAIDs and aspirin, however. Among these are that all NSAIDs as of 1984 can be bought only with a prescription (except ibuprofen), cost more than aspirin, cause fewer side effects in some people, and some are more convenient because they need to be taken only one or a few times per day.

As a group, the NSAIDs are similar in the way they are made, how safe they are, and how they work. Nevertheless, they appear to have subtle differences that cause some to work better than others for different kinds of arthritis and for different people. Some of the commonly used NSAIDs are listed in Table 2.

TABLE 2. A PARTIAL LIST OF PRESCRIPTION
NONSTEROIDAL ANTI-INFLAMMATORY DRUGS

Generic Name (Product Name)	Primary Uses
Choline magnesium trisalicylate (Trilisate)	Rheumatoid arthritis; osteoarthritis; certain other muscle/joint pain
Diflunisal (Dolobid)	Treatment of mild to moderate pain; osteoarthritis
Fenoprofen (Nalfon)	Rheumatoid arthritis; osteoarthritis; certain other joint/muscle pain
Ibuprofen (Motrin, Rufen)	Rheumatoid arthritis; osteoarthritis; certain other joint/muscle pain
Indomethacin (Indocin)	Ankylosing spondylitis; osteoarthritis; rheumatoid arthritis; acute gouty arthritis; certain other joint/muscle pain
Meclofenamate (Meclomen)	Rheumatoid arthritis; osteoarthritis; certain other joint/muscle pain
Mefenamic acid (Ponstel)	Short-term treatment of moderate pain

Generic Name (Product Name)	Primary Uses
Naproxen (Naprosyn)	Rheumatoid arthritis; osteoarthritis; certain other joint/muscle pain
Naproxen sodium (Anaprox)	Treatment of mild to moderate pain
Oxyphenbutazone (Tandearil)	Acute gouty arthritis; active rheumatoid arthritis; active ankylosing spondylitis
Phenylbutazone (Butazolidin)	Acute gouty arthritis; active rheumatoid arthritis; ankylosing spondylitis; painful shoulder; Reiter's syndrome
Piroxicam (Feldene)	Osteoarthritis; rheumatoid arthritis
Salsalate (Disalcid)	Rheumatoid arthritis; osteoarthritis; certain other muscle/joint pain
Sulindac (Clinoril)	Osteoarthritis; rheumatoid arthritis; ankylosing spondylitis; acute painful shoulder; acute gouty arthritis; certain other joint/muscle pain
Tolmetin (Tolectin)	Rheumatoid arthritis; juvenile arthritis; osteoarthritis; certain other joint/muscle pain
Zomepirac sodium (Zomax)	Moderate to severe pain

Possible Side Effects

The side effects associated with NSAIDs include nausea, vomiting, stomach pains and cramps, diarrhea or constipation, stomach bleeding, and ulcers. They may also include headaches, ringing in the ears, and blurred vision. They may also cause allergic-like symptoms in some people as can aspirin and should not be taken by people who develop asthma or nasal stuffiness from aspirin. A few doctors advise people taking NSAIDs to have regular tests of their blood and stool. This procedure helps them identify possible problems at an early stage, and permits them to consider changes in the drug therapy. As with all drugs, if any unusual effects show up, the doctor should be told.

The side effects of Oxyphenbutazone and phenylbutazone may be severe. Their use is ordinarily restricted to situations in which no other drug would do as well.

Corticosteroids

The corticosteroids (steroids for short) are man-made drugs that are related to cortisone and to hydrocortisone, the natural hormones made by the body's adrenal glands, which are located atop the kidneys. Specific steroid preparations in pill form include dexamethasone (Decadron, Dexone), prednisolone (Sterane, Delta-Cortef), prednisone (Deltasone, Orasone), hydrocortisone (A-hydroCort), triamcinolone (Aristocort), and betamethasone (Celestone).

Steroids are strong drugs and quickly reduce pain and inflammation. But although they relieve these symptoms effectively, they do not stop the underlying disease. They also may cause serious side effects, especially if used for months or years. As a result, corticosteroids are primarily given to people with severe arthritic disease (especially when vital organs are also involved) and for whom aspirin or other NSAIDs have not worked. Sometimes, however, they are used for short periods, especially during severe flare-ups. They are also occasionally given by injection directly into inflamed joints, a use that limits but does not prevent the chance that the person so treated will develop side effects. Injected corticosteroids relieve symptoms effectively, but usually do so only for a relatively short time. They carry a small risk that an infection may occur at the time of the injection.

Possible Side Effects

Steroids used for prolonged periods can cause mild side effects such as weight gain, rounding of the face, and easy bruising. They may also cause more serious side effects such as thinning of the bones, depression, high blood pressure, cataracts, muscle weakness, diabetes, an increased risk of infection, and rarely, bleeding from the stomach. No one person develops all of these side effects, and some occur only after high doses have been taken for months or years. If you experience any of these side effects, you should tell your doctor.

There are a few precautions for anyone who is taking steroids. These drugs slow down the adrenal glands. After some time, the glands reduce or stop making their own, natural steroids because they have been given signals by the pituitary gland located in the brain that the body already has enough of them. Yet when a person faces extra stress, such as that caused by surgery, infection, or major dental work, the body needs far more of these hormones than usual, and the adrenal glands of someone who is taking corticosteroids may not be able to make the extra amounts. If necessary, the only way to increase the amount of these hormones is for the doctor to raise the dosage temporarily until the stress period is over.

Because of these effects on the adrenal glands, if you are taking steroid drugs, you should inform all your physicians and dentists. Also, you should never decide on your own to stop or drastically reduce the amount of steroid drugs you are taking, even if you feel well. Your body won't be ready for weeks or even months to make its own hormones, and you may experience serious health problems. The cessation of corticosteroid treatment must be done slowly, with close supervision by a doctor.

Slow-Acting Drugs

Unlike the drugs described up to this point, another group may do more than just decrease inflammation and relieve symptoms. This group is known as the slow-acting, or disease-modifying, drugs. They are used primarily for treating rheumatoid arthritis in people for whom NSAIDs haven't been completely successful in controlling the disease. Many doctors believe that the slow-acting drugs may slow the underlying disease, though how they do this is not clear. This group of drugs includes gold, penicillamine, cytotoxic, and antimalarial drugs. All of the drugs in this group have to be taken for many weeks, and often for several months, before their full effects become noticeable. The relief they provide may last for some time after they are no longer being taken. But with these benefits of long-lasting relief and a possible slowing of the disease also comes a higher risk of serious side effects.

Gold Treatment

Injections of gold salts (gold sodium thiomalate, trade name Myochrysine, and aurothioglucose, trade name Solganol) have been used to treat rheumatoid arthritis for more than fifty years. For a long time, doctors were not sure how well they worked, but many studies have now shown that gold injections do help some people with rheumatoid arthritis who have not been helped by other drugs. The decision about whether to try gold—and when to begin if so—is not an easy one. It depends on how many and which joints are affected, how bad the symptoms are, the person's state of health, and how the joints appear on X-rays.

Once a decision is made to have a person try a gold salt, he or she will probably need to take gold for six to eight weeks or longer to learn if it will work. Relief comes gradually, if at all, during that time. Doctors sometimes prescribe other drugs to be taken with the gold treatment, especially in the early months before the gold has taken full effect. Eventually, some people can be taken off these other drugs if the gold works well for them.

A person stays on gold treatment for as long as it works, or until it produces side effects that require it to be stopped. These side effects may include skin rashes, damage to the kidneys and the bone marrow (particularly to the blood platelets that are produced there), and rarely, damage to the liver, lungs, or intestines. These effects usually go away once the drug has been stopped. People receiving gold therapy must have regular laboratory tests so that the less noticeable side effects of this treatment can be caught at an early stage.

To date, gold salts have been given only by injection, but gold tablets may eventually be on the market. These tablets seem to work almost as well as injected gold, and are expected to have fewer side effects. Gold injections have also been used successfully for juvenile arthritis and psoriatic arthritis.

Antimalarial Drugs

Antimalarial drugs (hydroxychloroquine sulfate, trade name Plaquenil) may be tried in the treatment of arthritis if other drugs have not worked. These drugs are related to quinine, and were originally used to treat malaria. They have since been found to reduce the symptoms and slow the disease process in some people with rheumatoid arthritis or systemic or discoid lupus erythematosus, although researchers have not fully understood how they work. Their full effects are often not felt for several months, if at all.

Although most people tolerate the antimalarial drugs well, a few will have the side effects of stomach upset or a skin rash. Muscle weakness is a rare side effect of these drugs. The most serious, but rare, side effect is damage to the retina of the eye, which can lead to blindness. Therefore, people taking antimalarial drugs must have regular eye examinations.

Penicillamine

As with the other slow-acting drugs, penicillamine is used for people with serious rheumatoid arthritis only after other medications have not been of help. It is available in tablets (Depen Titratabs) or capsules (Cuprimine). Although it is now being used only for rheumatoid arthritis, it is also being studied for use in treating scleroderma (see Chapter 13).

Penicillamine is not the same kind of drug as its distant cousin, penicillin, which is an antibiotic. For those in whom it works, it relieves joint pain, swelling, and stiffness after several months of therapy. Again, the side effects often require some people to stop taking this drug. Like gold, penicillamine may damage the kidneys and bone marrow, and may also cause fever, chills, rashes, sores in the mouth, a sore throat, stomach upset, muscle weakness, loss of taste, and easy bruising or bleeding. Because of these possible side effects, the drug is taken only with close supervision by a doctor, who will schedule laboratory tests to watch for these changes.

Cytotoxic Drugs

Cytotoxic drugs are potent medications that are used mainly to treat people with cancer and those who receive organ transplants. More recently, they have been used to treat people with serious rheumatoid arthritis, psoriatic arthritis, systemic lupus erythematosus, vasculitis, or polymyositis. Because the cytotoxic drugs are very potent, they are usually tried only after safer drugs have been shown to be of no help. Even then, doctors use them only for persons with severe disease, since their side effects are potentially dangerous and may outweigh their possible benefits.

The most commonly used cytotoxic drugs are azathioprine (Imuran), cyclophosphamide (Cytoxan), and methotrexate. These drugs reduce inflammation and seem to work at least partly by suppressing the immune system. As a result, the system becomes unable to carry out many of its functions, which is helpful to people with rheumatoid arthritis and systemic lupus erythematosus, since the immune system seems to be the major cause of damage to the body in these diseases. The cytotoxic drugs block the actions of the cells that make the abnormal antibodies in autoimmune diseases, and of those that are involved in inflammation. Unfortunately, these drugs also reduce the ability of the immune system to fight infections and otherwise protect the body from injury and disease.

Possible Side Effects

The side effects that may be caused by each of the cytotoxic drugs are different but include nausea, vomiting, diarrhea, and heartburn. People taking cytotoxic drugs may also have a higher risk of developing infection, skin rashes, easy bruising and bleeding, hair loss, blood in the urine or stool, ulcers, damage to the lungs, liver, or kidneys, and sterility. It is believed that the long-term use of azathioprine or cyclophosphamide creates a slight risk of the eventual development of cancer or leukemia. Because of these potential risks, doctors use the lowest possible dosage of a cytotoxic drug and schedule regular tests and checkups for anyone receiving such treatment.

SUMMARY

This chapter includes only some of the major drugs used in treating rheumatic diseases, particularly rheumatoid arthritis. Other drugs such as various pain-relievers and certain drugs used to control gout, are also useful (see Chapter 20). Some rheumatic diseases may cause systemic complications—such as eye inflammation—that require medications not described here.

Regardless of which medications you use, the important point is that they serve as one part of an overall treatment program.

CHAPTER SIX

Methods of Pain Control

To be successful at controlling pain, people with arthritis need to recognize that many factors influence the degree of their pain. For example, stress contributes to pain, as do fatigue and depression. If you are under much stress you may tense your muscles and have difficulty relaxing. Such tension increases the degree of pain that you experience. Likewise, if you're fatigued, your body may respond with increased pain because its tissues aren't getting the rest and repair they need. Depression feeds pain, often because you focus considerable attention on the pain itself rather than on more positive aspects of life. Pain, in turn, may feed each of these factors and increase their effect on you. The result may be a continuous cycle that is difficult to break. This cycle is sometimes referred to as the pain-stress-depression cycle.

Many people with arthritis find that they can control their pain by taking their medications on the schedule specified by their doctors, and by resting, exercising, keeping a positive attitude, and taking special care to protect their joints. Some, however, must use additional means for controlling their pain, especially during flare-ups of their disease. Fortunately, there are several effective ways to control pain, some of which have been around for years and others that are relatively new or experimental. Many pain-relieving techniques can be used at home; a few require visits to clinics for the use of special equipment. Doctors and other health professionals such as physical

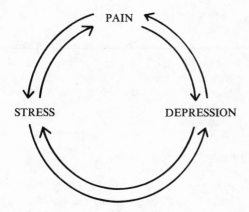

The pain-stress-depression cycle

or occupational therapists and some mental health workers help the person with arthritic pain to select and learn to use the appropriate methods.

Pain is the body's signal to rest an injured area, allow the tissues to be repaired, and prevent more harm from occurring. Therefore, you should not try to suppress pain with the goal of using your sore joints and muscles in the same way as you did before they became arthritic. If the pain is dulled and the affected area is used too soon or too hard, the damage and pain may continue. This cycle of pain and repeated damage may not be broken until enough rest is given to the affected area.

On the other hand, painful joints and muscles do have to be moved so that they don't become too stiff. Physicians sometimes suggest the use of a pain-control method just before daily exercise, so that the movements won't hurt too much and can be done as they should be. By working with your doctor or other health professional, you can learn to use pain-control methods to allow the right kinds of movement, such as proper exercise, while not allowing more harm to be done. The following descriptions are brief instructions for some pain-control techniques. People who think they might benefit from one or more of these methods should first ask their doctors or other health professionals for complete instructions about how to use them. Some of the methods can be dangerous if used incorrectly, or are useful only in certain situations.

HEAT TREATMENTS

The use of heat is an effective way to relax muscles and reduce the pain in arthritic joints. There are many ways to apply heat, some of which are best for small areas, such as the feet and hands, and others that heat large areas or the whole body.

Hot Baths and Showers

For people with many painful joints, doctors may recommend hot showers or baths, which help reduce stiffness by relaxing many muscles at the same time. Hot baths generally should last no longer than twenty minutes, after which they may cause fatigue. Whirlpool baths, with their moving water, are particularly pleasant. (People with certain disorders of the heart and blood vessels may have to avoid warm whirpool baths.) Large, warm pools are also helpful for people with very limited motion. The buoyancy of the water lets them do movements and gentle exercises that they can't do out of water.

Hot Compresses (Hydrocollator Packs)

Hot compresses help relieve pain in small areas of the body. To prepare these compresses, towels can be soaked in hot water, wrung out, and applied to the painful area. To hold heat in longer and protect the skin from burns, the hot towel should be covered with plastic sheets or dry towels. Hydrocollator packs contain silica gel, which retains heat for a long time. Heating these packs to the proper temperature, however, requires special equipment usually found only in a department of physical therapy.

Paraffin Wax Treatments

Another way to apply heat to the hands is with hot paraffin wax. The painful area is usually dipped ten to twelve times into a mixture of melted paraffin and oil, which then coats the area

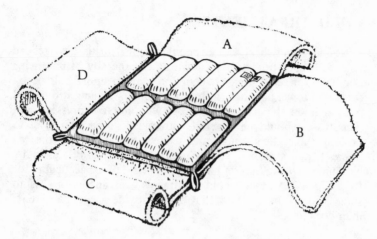

A hydrocollator pack

and keeps it warm for some time. The joints must remain in the same position once the process has begun or the wax will crack. After a period of fifteen to forty-five minutes, the wax is peeled off. This kind of treatment should not be used on parts of the body with open wounds.

Heat Lamps (Diathermy)

A heat lamp can be used to warm a small part of the body. It uses an infrared bulb (not an ultraviolet bulb as in a sun lamp) and is connected to an ordinary electrical outlet. The area to be treated is held about two feet from the bulb, and the treatment lasts approximately thirty minutes.

Heating Pads and Mitts

Electric heating pads are convenient, but are safe only if they are in good condition and used correctly. They are placed on top of the painful area for a short period. Heating pads should be used only at a low heat setting and only when you are fully awake. They should not be placed under the body. Electric mitts help to temporarily relieve sore hands.

COLD TREATMENTS

Besides using heat, some people with arthritis also relieve pain with cold treatments, known as cryotherapy, which helps numb the affected area. A common way to apply cold is by soaking a towel or other cloth in ice water, wringing it out, and putting it on the painful area. As with hot compresses, cold compresses should be covered with plastic or a dry towel to prolong their effectiveness and protect the skin from the extreme temperature. A cold compress can also be made by wrapping a towel around a plastic bag full of ice cubes or frozen peas. Although cold treatments feel uncomfortable to some people, others find that they provide more pain relief than does heat.

CONTRAST BATHS

Soaking the feet or hands alternately in a pail of hot water (110°F) for three minutes and one of cold water (65°F) for one minute provides excellent pain relief for many individuals.

MASSAGE

Some people with arthritis find that massage of the painful areas of their body provides relief. It helps relieve tension and provides warmth and relaxation to painful areas. You can massage yourself or have a partner help you. With experimentation, you can find the techniques that work best on certain areas. For example, deep, circular rubbing may help relieve a sore back, while a kneading motion may best help relieve a painful neck.

NEWER METHODS OF PAIN CONTROL

Although heat and cold treatments and massage are effective methods for relieving pain, newer methods may also prove useful. More physicians, physical and occupational therapists, and mental health workers now have a special interest in the control of chronic pain than was the case previously. These specialists are working to develop additional ways to break chronic cycles of pain.

Electrical Stimulation

A pain-control method that has recently been gaining popularity uses a device called a transcutaneous electrical nerve stimulator (TENS). The TENS unit consists of a generator with wire leads that have electrodes at the ends. A conducting gel is used to attach the electrodes to the skin near or on the area to be treated. When the unit is turned on, a low level of electricity is applied to the area. The person may feel a tingling sensation or nothing. The session may last from a few minutes

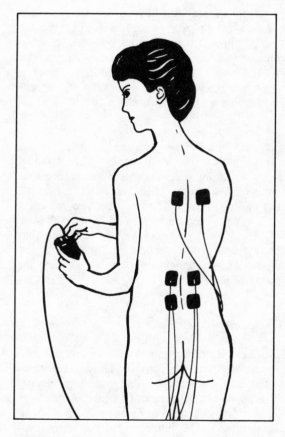

A TENS unit

to two hours, depending on the individual's needs and the treatment prescription. TENS units range in size from small, portable ones about the size of a flashlight to the larger units used in hospitals. Some people with arthritis have gotten pain relief from TENS treatment; others have not. The relief may last from a few hours to days. Since a TENS unit costs $150 or more, before buying you should rent one for a month or more to see if it provides relief. The benefit from TENS usually diminishes with the passage of time.

Relaxation Techniques

Besides TENS treatment and the other methods described above, pain specialists are testing various ways of teaching people how to relax. Pain is often increased by tense muscles, and relaxation helps people loosen these muscles and think less about their pain. Methods of relaxation include meditation, hypnosis, and self-hypnosis. Some involve learning to concentrate on pleasant thoughts and on doing deep breathing exercises.

Some specialists teach people to relax through biofeedback training. With this kind of training, you can learn to control some automatic functions of your body—such as blood flow or brain activity—by watching or listening to various measurements, such as brain waves shown on a screen or a beeping sound that matches the heart beat. With practice, you can learn to slow down or change the measurement, and as a result, you may feel more relaxed. Thus far, experiments have shown that this kind of training helps people reduce pain from migraine and tension headaches, but whether or not it works well for the pain of chronic arthritis is less clear.

Behavior Modification

Some pain researchers are trying to help people control pain by getting them to change certain behaviors. These researchers use a method called behavior modification that helps people limit the effect of pain on their actions. The method involves encouraging and rewarding talk or actions not related to pain, such as talk about politics or beginning a hobby. It involves disapproval or ignoring of any complaints of pain, and family members are instructed to do the same at home. After some time, a person in a behavior modification program will realize that the talk of pain just leads to pain, whereas showing other interests leads to pleasant rewards such as enthusiasm and attention from others. In this way, pain stops being the center of behavior and becomes just one part of the person's life.

The methods described above for relieving pain should be tried only under the supervision of a physician or other appropriate health professional. Many people seeking relief from pain have fallen for false claims for drugs or devices that promise to "eliminate" pain (see Chapter 9). Many unscrupulous promoters take advantage of people with chronic pain and use powerful arguments to get them to purchase questionable treatments. To avoid such traps, people with arthritis are advised to check with their doctors before trying anything to treat their symptoms. Qualified pain specialists are available to help, but often provide care only to people referred to them by other doctors.

Controlling pain is an important part of treatment for many people with arthritis. Remember, however, that the most effective control of pain is usually achieved by following a combination of several different forms of treatment recommended by your doctor and other health workers. Medications, rest, proper exercise, a positive mental attitude, and the careful use of arthritic joints will go far toward helping reduce chronic pain and breaking the pain-stress-depression cycle. Additional pain-control methods can be useful supplements to this balanced program.

CHAPTER SEVEN

Surgery

Most people with arthritis can control their disease with proper physical therapy, medications, rest, and proper use of their joints. Sometimes, though, severe arthritis causes enough damage to the joints and other tissues that surgery may be needed. The surgical procedures and rehabilitative techniques used in treating badly damaged joints have become very successful. Both continue to improve as physicians learn more about arthritis and refine and develop their surgical techniques.

The person with arthritis should never rush into surgery. Except for infectious arthritis (see Chapter 20), arthritis seldom poses an emergency, and any surgery should therefore be carefully considered before a decision is made. In most cases, physicians recommend that medical treatments be exhausted before surgery is undertaken. Surgery for some forms of arthritis is considered only after a long period in which other treatments such as physical therapy and drug therapy and modifications of your lifestyle have been tried; in other conditions, however, early surgery may help prevent extensive damage to the joints.

No one should have surgery until he or she has a clear idea of its possible benefits and complications. By understanding what surgery can and can't do in a particular situation, you will be better able to reach the proper decision. There are few hard-and-fast rules on the timing of non-emergency surgery ("elective" surgery). Even the choice of the best surgical procedure for a given situation can be difficult, because of continual progress and change.

Obtaining an opinion from a second surgeon will often help you learn more about the pros and cons of surgery in your situation. A difference in opinion between surgeons does not necessarily indicate that one is right and the other wrong; the situation may be one in which treatment is debatable, or in which several different procedures would produce similar results when done by experienced surgeons.

How do you choose a surgeon? The best place to start is to ask your physician for a referral to a surgeon who has extensive experience in the type of surgery you may need. Some surgeons have particular experience with specific operations and conditions. Having evaluated individuals with similar problems, they are best able to advise you whether surgery is appropriate, and if indicated, which procedure is best for you. They can also explain your role in the rehabilitative program following surgery.

POSSIBLE REASONS FOR SURGERY

There are several reasons for considering joint surgery. In arthritis (primarily rheumatoid arthritis and osteoarthritis), the wearing away of joint cartilage may cause the joints to become stiff, painful, or unstable. When this damage is extensive, severe or constant pain, loss of function, and deformity can result. When the disease damages a tendon, the involved joint may be immobilized. Involvement of the weight-bearing joints such as the hips, knees, or ankles may seriously interfere with your ability to walk, while involvement of the upper extremities may limit your ability to perform even the simple activities of daily living. Thus, except when surgery is performed to prevent future damage, the indications for surgery are pain (when it can't be reduced by rest, heat and cold therapy, prescribed exercise, splinting, or medication), deformity, and loss of function.

What benefits should you expect from surgery? This, of course, depends on the degree of damage and the surgery performed. Relief of pain is the most likely outcome. Your surgeon would be able to tell you what benefits you can expect, but also what limitations are inherent in a procedure. Improvements in movement and function are usual but are less predictable. Surgery may help considerably for someone with constant hip pain or limitation of motion that interferes with sexual enjoyment. In some types of surgery, such as replacement of the knuckle joint in the hand, people can expect that the hand's cosmetic apearance will be improved. Although arthritis surgery is not indicated for purely cosmetic reasons, a better-looking, more normal limb is certainly a positive result. Your family physician and surgeon can advise you how much relief of pain and improvement in function or appearance is likely. You and you alone must then decide whether the benefits are worth the surgery.

Part of the decision or timing may depend on the costs and on how much of these costs will be covered by your health insurance—or, for those who qualify, by Medicaid or Medicare. To avoid unwelcome surprises, it is important to check into your coverage before undergoing surgery, and to discuss the expected costs with your surgeons.

REASONS NOT TO HAVE SURGERY

Your family physician or rheumatologist, in consultation with a surgeon, may explain that surgery for your particular condition will not sufficiently relieve pain, improve function, or result in a better physical appearance. If so, these are clear reasons not to have surgery. Even if surgical treatment could be expected to help, other reasons must also be considered in the matter of avoiding an operation. Before considering any surgery, you should undergo a thorough evaluation by your family physician to determine whether you are an appropriate candidate. Thus, for example, surgery poses a high risk for the person with serious heart or lung disease, since it is a strain on even the healthiest person. Since surgery for the effects of arthritis is elective, other health problems should be under as much control, as possible before the operation is performed.

A person's age is an important consideration is deciding whether to have joint replacement surgery. Since an artificial joint may loosen in time, the younger a person is at the time of surgery, the more likely he or she is to eventually have to undergo further surgery. Also, younger people are more physically active than older people, and put more stress on a surgically treated joint, making it more likely to break down or loosen.

People who are overweight have an increased rate of complications. Obesity puts extra stress on the heart and lungs. It may also hinder the recovery of a weight-bearing joint (such as a hip or knee) if surgery is done on such a joint. Too much body weight puts added pressure on the tissues undergoing repair and may interfere with the rehabilitation necessary for recovery. Obese persons may be advised to reduce their weight before surgery.

You must be realistic about what to expect from surgery. Although the doctor cannot possibly predict its exact results, there are certain limits to what it can achieve.

One possible complication of surgery is an infection in the wound. To reduce the risk of this, any bacterial infections already present in the body before surgery must be cleared up before the operation is performed. Otherwise, they may spread to the treated area and cause serious damage. A postoperative infection may occur even if the person undergoing surgery had not been infected before his or her operation. In some operations, the risk of infection has been reduced in recent years by more rigorous sterile technique in operating rooms, and the use of antibiotics at the time of surgery. Nonetheless, the risk has not been eliminated.

Before you decide to have surgery, you must also accept the fact that afterwards you will have to follow a strict treatment and rehabilitation plan. Unlike surgery for the removal of a diseased organ, such as an appendix, the optimal results of arthritis surgery depend to a large extent on the patient's participation in his or her care. The operation is only the first step toward restoring a joint. After the surgery is done, the amount of work you put into the recovery process can make the difference between success and failure. Because rehabilitation after surgery is so vitally important to the outcome of surgery, someone who doesn't intend to or can't manage to follow the surgeon's recommendations may be better off *not* going through the expense and pain involved in a surgical operation.

KINDS OF JOINT SURGERY

There are several different kinds of surgery for arthritis. Each operation is planned to correct a specific problem. To better understand the kinds of operations available, review the structures of the joints described in Chapter 2.

A relatively recent surgical advance is arthroscopy, the use of a small periscope to see into a joint, most commonly the knee. The arthroscope, which is a bit larger than a drinking straw, enables a surgeon to see virtually everything inside the knee. The doctor can look directly into the joint or view an image projected onto a television screen. The arthroscope can also be moved around inside the joint to provide the doctor with different views of the tissues. It is a valuable aid in diagnosing knee injuries and assessing joint damage from arthritis.

Surgery can also be performed right through the arthroscope via a separate small hole, using special microscopic tools. With this technique the doctor can shave or remove bits of torn or loose cartilage. The procedure, which generally requires full anesthesia, leaves only small puncture wounds rather than large surgical scars, thus permitting more rapid rehabilitation. The risk of infection is also reduced. Arthroscopy is used primarily on the knee, but is also performed on the shoulder and hip.

Another type of operation done for arthritis is known as a synovectomy. This procedure is done to remove part or all of a diseased or excessive synovial membrane ("syno" refers to synovium; "ectomy" = surgical removal of). In some forms of arthritis, especially rheumatoid arthritis, the synovium becomes inflamed. This inflammation leads to enlargement or thickening of the synovium and the release of enzymes which, over the years, damage the cartilage, tendon, ligament, and bone of the affected joints. Pain and swelling may be persistent. A synovectomy is one way to reduce these effects, but the synovium usually grows back after surgery and, with it, the pain and swelling usually return. A synovectomy is now performed primarily to prevent tendons from eroding and only rarely to remove synovium from the joints.

An operation called an osteotomy is done to correct a joint deformity by cutting and then resetting a bone in its proper alignment ("osteo" = bone; "otomy" = surgical cutting). Osteotomies are useful if the cartilage is worn away more on one side of the end of a bone than on the other, causing misalignment at the joint. This change allows the weight to be placed on the relatively normal part of a joint.

A resection is an operation in which the surgeon removes all or part of a bone. It is done in places where experience has shown that the body can function with minimal pain without the joint. It is sometimes done because the joints in the middle parts of the feet have become deformed making walking extremely painful and difficult. Painful bunions (swellings at the base of the big toe that push the toe outwards) can also be removed by resection.

An operation known as arthrodesis, or bone fusion, is done to relieve extreme pain in joints whose motion can be sacrificed —usually in the ankles or wrists. In this surgery, the bones at the joint are cut so they fit together. The bones are held rigidly in place so that the joint will fuse, and the joint is "frozen" in place. Although the joint loses flexibility, it can support weight easily and without pain.

Many people have heard of the rebuilding of damaged joints, a procedure called arthroplasty (arth = joint, plasty = surgical formation of, or shaping). This is done by resurfacing or re-lining the ends of those bones whose cartilage has worn away, with the bone or ligaments being damaged as a result. Arthro-plasty also refers to the replacement of an entire joint with an artificial joint made of plastic and metal. This procedure has revolutionized the field of arthritis surgery. Total joint replace-ment has been used widely for about twenty years, and the results have been generally excellent. The most successful and frequent joint replacement operations are for the hip, knuckles, and the knee. Shoulder replacement is fairly successful, while wrist and ankle replacement are still experimental.

JOINTS THAT MIGHT BENEFIT FROM SURGERY

Hand and Wrist

Losing the function of the hands or wrists, especially when there is also pain in these joints, can be a serious matter. Some people may also be embarrassed by the appearance of deformed hands. When other therapy has not allowed someone with such difficulties to do necessary tasks such as holding a fork or closing or opening zippers, surgery may be indicated. Most hand surgery is performed for three reasons: better function, less pain, and improved appearance.

Several kinds of surgery may be done on the hands and wrists. The procedure chosen depends on which bones and joints and tendons are involved and the extent of the damage. Synovectomy is sometimes done for the joints of the wrists, mainly in the early stages of arthritis, before deformity becomes a major problem. If the wrist is severely painful or badly mis-shapen, several procedures are considered. Fusion (or arthro-desis) limits the extent to which the wrist can move, but when successul relieves pain dramatically and makes the hand more stable. Resection of the end of one or more of the bones in the wrist (or removal of all the wrist bones) may improve the motion of this joint and reduce pain in it. Total joint replace-ment is another possibility for a damaged wrist, but is not recommended for someone who will be doing heavy labor using the wrist.

Because deformity of the hands does not always cause them to lose their function, surgery may not be needed for this reason alone. However, when the hand is also very painful and is not helped by more basic treatments, the finger joints (espe-cially those at the junction of the fingers and palm) may be replaced with silicone rubber implants. This procedure is usually successful in providing pain relief and a better appearance of the hands. As for other artificial joints, months of follow-up physical therapy are required to achieve good function.

In 1983, some 10,000 people with arthritis, most of whom have disfiguring rheumatoid arthritis, had diseased joints in their

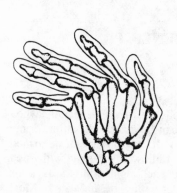 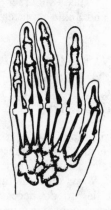

HAND BEFORE JOINT REPLACEMENT SURGERY

HAND AFTER FINGER JOINT REPLACEMENTS

Finger joint replacement

hands replaced with tiny Silastic "hinges," which rely on muscle tension and surrounding tissues for support. These hinges can produce some cosmetic and functional improvement, particularly in the proximal (knuckle) joints.

People with hands that have been badly affected by rheumatoid arthritis may also develop dorsal tenosynovitis, a complication that affects the long tendons on the back of the hand ("dorsal" = back; "teno" = tenon; "synovitis" = inflammation of the synovial membrane). The tendons on the palm side may also be affected, but less frequently. This condition produces a soft mass that does not itself hurt but makes the hand hurt. Occasionally, the tissue is removed surgically to prevent damage to and eventual rupture of the tendons. Nevertheless, an affected tendon sometimes tears and must be repaired. This tearing is usually painless, but can be recognized by sudden loss of the ability to extend (straighten) a finger at the knuckle joint. If done early, the surgery for repairing this condition is relatively simple and usually successful. The person normally recovers within a few weeks, although splinting is necessary to protect the tendon from excessive pull until it is adequately repaired. Sometimes surgery is done to re-align the tendons to improve movement of the fingers and hand, especially if the fingers flare outward.

The Hip

Some people with arthritis in a hip face constant pain and have difficulty walking, sitting, and standing. Many such people can now be helped dramatically through hip-replacement surgery. The total relief of pain and restored hip function have been the results for thousands of people. In 1983 alone, over 150,000 Americans had a total hip replacement. The short-term success rate in hip-replacement surgery is 95 percent in osteoarthritis and almost as high in rheumatoid arthritis.

In deciding the timing and type of surgical procedure to be done on a diseased hip, the condition of the bones and the age of the person are considered. Formerly, hip replacement was done only on people over age 45 because eventually the artificial joint was likely to slip. The cement now used for anchoring a hip replacement can be expected to stay intact for many years, although loosening may still be a problem. Progress in

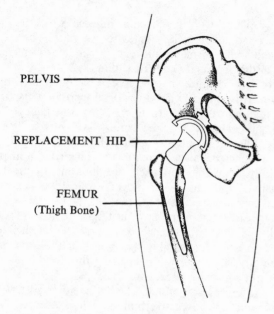

Total hip joint replacement

design and technique has made hip replacement possible in younger people, though some still have to have artificial hips replaced a second or third time because of loosening.

Some of the problems of hip-replacement loosening may be circumvented with "porous ingrowth," an experimental process whereby specialists try to get the person's own bone to grow directly into and fuse with the microscopic pores of the metal part of the hip replacement to form a longer-lasting connection. Hundreds of such operations have proven successful over the short term since surgeons began doing them, but only time will determine whether this procedure will prove more durable than the use of cement in hip replacements.

A cementless hip replacement that is screwed, not glued, into place is being tested in people under age fifty with arthritis. So far people who have had this procedure have done well, but it will probably require another ten years to assess the value of this and similar techniques.

An alternative to total replacement is hip resurfacing, which is usually just as effective in relieving pain, but probably will not last as long as a complete replacement. In this operation the diseased part of the top of the thigh bone is cleaned away and capped with a metal covering. At the same time, the socket of the hip is cleaned and lined with plastic. Whether this procedure has an effect that lasts as long or is as effective as total joint replacemnet is debatable, and the procedure is therefore seldom done anymore.

New materials for hip replacements are also being tried. In some cases, publicity in the newspapers report dramatic breakthroughs. However, adequate study has not yet been performed to evaluate the long-term effects of a new design. Many designs which originally looked promising were failures in years to follow.

The Shoulder

Shoulders affected with arthritis are sometimes helped by synovectomy if exercise, heat, cold, medicine, and steroid injections have not reduced the pain in these joints. However, while complete replacement of the shoulder joint usually relieves pain, it restores only some of the movement. The operation is difficult, and only a few surgeons have had extensive experience with shoulder arthroplasties. The person who has such surgery usually needs many months to recover.

Ankle and Foot

A person with arthritis can be seriously limited by pain in the ankle or foot and by deformity of the toes. These structures bear all of the body's weight. If the use of orthotics and special shoes does not help the person get around, surgery should be considered. A deformed foot should not undergo surgery unless it is bothering you or unless the skin is breaking down and causing infections.

Many surgical procedures can be performed for arthritis in the joints of the feet. Fusion of the bones at the back of the foot or ankle is one of the most common of these procedures. Replacement of the ankle is now being done only experimentally. Sometimes the ends of the bones in the arch and the toes are removed when pain in that part of the foot prevents walking or is causing pressure sores and infections. Also, toe deformities can be corrected by resection, cutting away bone, fusion, or replacement of toe joints.

The Knee

The knee is potentially a relatively unstable joint on which life-long, heavy demands are made. It is particularly susceptible to injury because of its exposed position and the stress it must bear. If arthritis in the knee has not responded well to non-surgical therapy, your orthopedic surgeon may suggest surgery. Many different types of surgery are available depending on the disease, your age, the extent of damage, associated problems and the desired results. About 150,000 knee joints are replaced annually. As with total hip replacement, porous ingrowth is being tested to see if it will solve the problem of joint loosening.

The Elbow

The person with arthritis of the elbow may elect surgery to relieve pain, restore motion, or both. A painful or unstable elbow can severely limit the use of the wrist and hand. Synovectomy, with or without resection, can provide pain relief if the pain is caused by an inflamed synovial membrane, but not if it is the result of degenerative arthritis or injury to the elbow. If the elbow has limited movement, resurfacing or joint re-

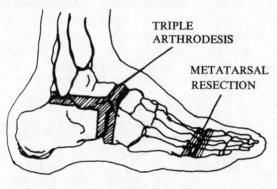

TRIPLE
ARTHRODESIS

METATARSAL
RESECTION

Two types of foot surgery

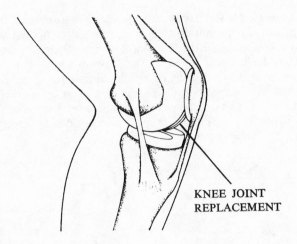

KNEE JOINT
REPLACEMENT

Knee joint replacement

placement may be advised. Elbow joint replacement is not as successful as hip replacement, because of the propensity for dislocation. One new model, the Capitello-Condylar elbow, is currently under investigation, and the early results appear promising, since it seems to dislocate less frequently than older models. The typical recipient is the older patient over seventy.

AFTER SURGERY

Your surgeon will prescribe a specific program of rest, physical therapy, and limited activity following surgery. Before deciding to have surgery, you need to be sure that your household can be arranged to facilitate your full recovery. After surgery, many people need days or weeks of rest and must use splints, canes, or crutches to perform their usual tasks. Most will have a special exercise routine for regaining the strength and mobility of their repaired joint(s). Each person should discuss with his or her surgeon what short-term limitations to expect and what role he or she should take in the recovery period. This permits plans to be made ahead of time, and a smooth recovery.

Surgery for arthritis, while not a cure, can be an important part of the overall treatment program and can lead to improved

79

movement and a better quality of life. No treatment, whether drug, surgery, or physical therapy, can fully succeed without the wholehearted participation of the person being treated. The combined efforts of the entire health-care team—the doctors, nurses, physical therapists, occupational therapists, social workers, and most important, the person with arthritis—are essential to success. Collaboration among and between these team members is particularly important for those considering surgery.

CHAPTER EIGHT

Living with Arthritis

Living with any chronic disease can be difficult. For some people, arthritis disrupts family life, work, sexuality, relations with friends, finances, and the tasks of everyday living. For others, it is mild, only slightly affecting their activities and emotions.

Taking care of the social and emotional effects of arthritis is just as important as treating its physical effects. Treatment of these aspects, however, cannot begin until any problems are recognized, brought out in the open, and met head on. Fortunately, there are people and places to turn to for help. Many agencies, organized services, and community groups can and will help people with arthritis work to solve emotional, financial, and practical problems caused by their illness. But because these groups cannot possibly seek out all those who need their help, the person with arthritis must take the initiative and find out where to go for assistance.

Your first step is to ask for help in locating such services. Physicians, nurses, social workers, and other health-care professionals may be able to help directly or refer you to others who can. The chapters of the Arthritis Foundation (see Chapter 26) help people find services in their local areas. Another starting point is the local community council, health and welfare council, or council of social agencies. Such agencies, under various names, are found in most communities and can help you get in touch with the right health and social-service agencies.

EMOTIONAL EFFECTS

The overall effect of arthritis on the person who has it, and on his or her family, is decided in part by the type and severity of the disease. A major part of handling the problems arthritis can create depends on how determined you are to overcome its effects. Your attitude largely decides whether the disease will turn into a personal disaster or a manageable situation.

Just as you must learn to overcome the physical problems of pain, fatigue, inflammation, and stiff joints, you must actively learn to understand and then deal with the emotional and social difficulties they can cause. It takes time, effort, and considerable patience to rise above arthritis. There are many hurdles to overcome, largely caused by the nature of rheumatic diseases themselves. People with arthritis feel discomfort and pain. Some often feel tired and experience difficulty with maneuvers they were once easily able to do. Moreover, the symptoms of arthritis increase and subside without warning, leading many people to hesitate when making plans for future activities.

No wonder many people with arthritis have a hard time adjusting emotionally to their new situations. Some people react by feeling depressed, angry, or frustrated by their new limitations and by the unpredictable nature of their symptoms. Many, fearing or questioning what the future may hold, may lose some of their self-confidence, and question their previous self-image. Some people have described feeling overwhelmed by all of the problems posed by arthritis.

The emotional effects of rheumatic disease cannot be separated from the physical ones. Although emotions don't cause or cure the symptoms of arthritis, they can have a profound effect on these symptoms. As mentioned earlier, some people get locked into a vicious cycle that starts with pain, which leads them to feel depressed. Their depression makes them tense, causing them to lose sleep and to focus more attention on their pain, fatigue, and other stresses they have. The fatigue and increased tension cause still more pain, which feeds the cycle all over again. Further difficulty in any aspect of the cycle aggravates the difficulty in the others. A person can become trapped in the negative cycle and may need help to break out of it.

Some people react to these emotions and pain by withdrawing into themselves and shutting out their families and friends in an effort to ignore the physical and emotional effects of their disease. Such denial is a normal reaction, as are anger, frustration, fear, and depression. These reactions, however, keep people from accepting the reality of their arthritis, and from learning to make the most of their lives. The cycle won't be broken until the affected person makes a conscious effort to do so.

It can be done. Each aspect of the cycle must be identified and addressed in turn. Earlier chapters have presented ideas on how to control pain, fatigue, and stress. The first step in controlling a negative emotional outlook is to recognize all of one's thoughts and feelings and to get them out in the open. People need to tell those close to them—their friends, families, doctors, nurses, and some work associates—how their diseases affect them. Such open discussions help those with arthritis to share their frustrations with others and learn to accept their diseases. This doesn't mean becoming resigned to an illness; rather, it helps you understand what to expect, learn to work around limitations, and have a realistic outlook on the effects of arthritis. People who do accept their arthritis are more apt to follow all aspects of their treatment programs because they recognize the need for treatment. They control the physical effects of their ailment, which helps them uncover and learn to control the emotional effects as well.

Open discussions about the effects of arthritis are also valuable because they help friends and relatives to understand the actions and needs of the person with arthritis. Many people have misconceptions about arthritis, thinking that it brings only minor problems. Unless they are told of its true effects, they may misinterpret the changing reactions of someone with a fluctuating rheumatic disease as the actions of a finicky person asking for attention.

Some people find it difficult, especially at first, to discuss their emotions with those close to them. In such situations, talks with other sympathetic listeners may help them learn to better communicate their thoughts. A variety of understanding professional people are available to listen and help the person with arthritis solve personal, financial, and family problems. For example, church members may want to discuss their concerns with members of their clergy. Others may meet with psychologists, personal counselors, or social workers affiliated with family-service agencies. These professionals help people to reach their own decisions and to find other sources of help.

In many communities, people with arthritis have formed

arthritis clubs or support groups in which they discuss mutual problems and share solutions with others who know just how they feel. These clubs help them to realize that they are not alone in their difficulties. They also introduce persons with rheumatic diseases to others who have learned to overcome various types of such disease and to lead full lives. These people can provide a powerful motivation to others struggling to take charge of their lives. (See Appendix A for a listing of helpful agencies and organizations.)

As emphasized in earlier chapters, taking responsibility for self-care is crucial for the person with arthritis. From a medical standpoint, a treatment program is optimal only if it is followed diligently. Such self-discipline is also important from a psychological viewpoint. As the person becomes aware of the benefits of controlling the physical effects of arthritis, he or she feels more in control of the situation. The cycle of pain, depression, and stress is more easily broken, and persons who practice self-care will come to understand the strong influence they have on their own emotions.

ARTHRITIS AND SEXUAL PROBLEMS

Although arthritis almost never affects the genitals, it may have an indirect effect on a person's sexuality. It can cause stiffness, pain, tiredness, and self-consciousness from the physical changes it produces. Hip problems, particularly, can interfere with sexual activity in some people. By initiating sex, your partner may also feel awkward and fearful of causing you more pain. These problems may lead to decreased enjoyment of sex and possibly to major personal and family problems.

Arthritis can cause changes in the joints and other body parts that can alter how a person looks and moves. If you allow it, these changes can interfere with an otherwise healthy self-image by causing you to feel less feminine or masculine, less youthful, or less confident sexually or socially. It is possible, but sometimes hard, to work through these negative emotions—the person with arthritis can come to accept the changes it causes and yet maintain his or her personal interests in life.

As is true for overcoming the other emotional effects of arthritis, the first step toward treating sexual problems is to acknowledge and discuss them. Sexual problems are particularly difficult for some people to talk about, but if ignored, minor difficulties or anxieties may become major and disrupt important relationships.

Open lines of communication, both with your sexual partner and with your physician or other health professional will go a long way toward easing difficult situations. Talking about the anxieties, fears, hopes, and practical sexual problems posed by your arthritis will help you find solutions and maintain a fulfilling sexual relationship. Frequently, however, neither your physician nor your partner will bring up the topic, so you must often take the initiative. Once the subject is broached, further discussions should come more easily.

It is important and realistic for people with arthritis to know that help is available for solving sexual problems that it may create. Individual health professionals can provide counseling themselves or refer those who come to them to others specially trained to help with sexual problems. These counselors can suggest how you can be open and honest with your partner so that you both can enjoy a satisfying sexual relationship despite your arthritis. They can also recommend certain positions that put less stress on your diseased joints. These are problems for which there are solutions; even people with severe disabilities can have fulfilling sexual lives.

FINANCIAL PROBLEMS

Rheumatic diseases often pose a significant financial drain on those who develop them. Just how much of a drain depends on how severe the symptoms are, on what special treatment the person needs, and on the person's type of employment. Medical costs can accumulate from doctor visits, laboratory tests, physical or occupational therapy, medication, surgery, self-help devices, transportation to treatment centers, aids such as splints or canes, counseling sessions, and the use of homemaker services. The family that was once on solid financial ground may find its resources depleted by such costs.

Few families can carry such burdens alone. For some people, the medical costs of arthritis are partly covered by health insurance through their employers or private insurance policies. Some states have established by law high-risk health insurance pools that make such insurance available to anyone, regardless of health status. Unfortunately, such policies are very expensive. Others are eligible for benefits under Medicare (for which eligibility is determined by age, chronic disability, or both), under Medicaid (with benefits, based on income, that vary from state to state), or under Social Security Disability Insurance. Children with arthritis are eligible for assistance with educational and medical problems through Crippled Children's Services, the Developmental Disabilities Act, and under Public Law 94-142. Other kinds of financial help vary greatly in different communities. One source of financial help may be the state Department of Social Service (or Department of Welfare), which sometimes provides emergency assistance. For these public programs, the individual with arthritis must usually apply in person, and the procedures can be frustratingly slow.

The local chapters of the Arthritis Foundation provide guidance for those who need help in learning about the benefits for which they may qualify and how to apply for them. Physicians, nurses, or workers at medical clinics may refer people with arthritis to social workers trained to help them find the right assistance.

ARTHRITIS AND WORK

For many people, financial security means the ability to work and earn a living. If this ability is threatened by arthritis, there is cause for concern, but not for despair. Employers are not required by law to make any special provisions for workers who have difficulty performing their tasks because of arthritis or any other chronic illness. Nonetheless, most companies are anxious to retain the services of trained employees. A few simple adjustments in working conditions may be all that are needed to enable someone with arthritis to continue his or her occupation. A new chair, a desk of the correct height, shop tools placed at a more convenient level, or allowance for short rest periods during the day are some of the ways used to reduce strain and fatigue and accommodate limited motion. If these adjustments are not enough, a transfer to another position within the company—one better suited to the person's abilities —may be possible. Such transfers may be difficult if the new position requires much retraining or disrupts an established seniority system within a department. A shift in working hours to avoid spending time in heavy traffic may also help people who are easily fatigued.

Just how to request these changes depends on the attitude of the employer. It is usually best to begin by talking with your foreman, personnel director, or union steward.

People with arthritis who need help in finding or choosing a suitable job should contact their State Employment Services. These services are available without charge, and workers in the Selective Placement units are often knowledgeable about job placement and careers for disabled persons.

Some people with arthritis will eventually be unable to continue the occupations in which they are trained and experienced, and will have to seek different vocations. Questions about job retraining can be answered by the Department of Vocational Rehabilitation, an agency operated by each state to help disabled people with employment difficulties. The Department of Vocational Rehabilitation provides thorough medical examinations, aptitude tests to measure employment abilities, and interviews to clarify each person's working potential. On the basis of this information, the Department, if it accepts an individual for services, recommends a vocational training program that will be paid for with state funds. Unfortunately, vocational rehabilitation departments accept relatively few people with arthritis for such training. Although the actual job placement record for people with arthritis who are accepted into the program is quite good, a prejudice exists that people with arthritis are poor risks for job training. The reasons appear to be mainly the fluctuating course of many forms of arthritis and the complex patterns of joint involvement that vary among individuals and make it difficult to classify work limitations precisely. The Arthritis Foundation is currently engaged in a cooperative venture with the Rehabilitation Services Administration, which is responsible for vocational rehabilitation, to overcome these problems.

DISABILITY BENEFITS

People whose arthritis has left them unable to work in gainful employment may be eligible for certain disability benefits. The term "disability benefits" has many legal meanings. Each person may need to make several inquiries (because of new and changing legislation or insurance company rules) to find out what help is available for his or her particular situation.

In some states, employers must carry insurance to compensate their employees for the temporary loss of wages caused by illnesses not related to work. Those who believe they are temporarily unable to work should ask their personnel officers or union representatives whether they are eligible for such disability benefits. Those who are covered by their own group health insurance plans should examine their policies for workloss benefits.

Long-term disability benefits are provided by the federal Social Security Administration. People who cannot continue working may be eligible for Social Security Disability Insurance or Supplemental Security Income disability benefits. Both require that the disabling condition lasts or is expected to last continuously for at least twelve months. You and your physician must provide detailed information about your medical situation so that the Social Security Administration can decide whether you are eligible for these benefits.

Social Security Disability Insurance is funded through taxes paid by workers and employers to the Social Security Trust Fund. The benefits do not start until the beginning of the sixth month after a worker has become disabled. After the sixth month, the first check will include any back payments. To qualify for such benefits, you must have held a job in which you made contributions to the Social Security Trust Fund for a specified number of years, depending on your age and the year in which your disability began. Certain family members of a worker who has become disabled may also be eligible for such payments. The rules for eligibility can be obtained from any Social Security office.

Supplemental Security Income was the first federal cash assistance program in this country for the general public. It is designed to provide a floor of income for aged, blind, or otherwise disabled people who have little or no income or other financial resources. There are strict income limits for eligibility under this program. In contrast to Disability Insurance, the Supplemental Security program is supported through general tax funds and not through the special taxes (FICA) withheld from paychecks for the Social Security Trust Fund.

States may add their own payments to federal Supplemental Security Income benefits, and no waiting period is required before the benefits begin. No back payments are made. A person whose financial resources are lower than a certain level can receive Supplemental Security Income benefits during the waiting period for Disability Insurance and still be eligible for both kinds of benefits.

The Arthritis Foundation and its divisions and chapters have prepared a guide to Social Security disability programs for people with arthritis. If you think you may be eligible, visit or call your local Social Security offices. The workers there can help you obtain proper medical information from your doctors or clinics, and explain the benefits you may receive.

HELP AT HOME

In some situations, people with arthritis may need nursing services or housekeeping help at home. For example, some people need extra help with shopping, cooking, cleaning, and child care during flare-ups of their disease or before or after they enter a hospital. Such situations are usually temporary, and can often be handled by getting a part-time housekeeper for a few weeks or months. It is also often possible to obtain a homemaker with special training in managing a household in which someone is ill or convalescing. Additionally, some communities offer a "Meals on Wheels" service to help in emergencies. The local family service agency or local Arthritis Foundation chapter can help you find such services.

If you are homebound, your physician may recommend that you get regular nursing care or physical therapy. Some communities have visiting nurse and public health nursing agencies to provide at-home help to people whose physicians request these services. The nurses who come from these agencies will provide home professional care and teach your family members how to provide such care between the nurses' visits. Some agencies also have physical therapists who can demonstrate proper exercises at home and teach families how to assist the person with arthritis.

People who are homebound and spend long periods alone may benefit from a "Friendly Visitor" program. Many Arthritis Foundation chapters, churches, and other local groups offer these services, in which the homebound person receives regular visits from someone in the local area. Often, people with arthritis or related diseases who have received special training about the disease and community resources are available to help others with rheumatic diseases. Beyond this, the person with arthritis can often find willing visitors informally, simply by asking neighbors, relatives, and friends for someone who'd be happy for companionship. Such visits distract the homebound person from his or her pain or depression and help that person to feel more motivated toward self care. They also provide valuable contact with the community and reduce feelings of isolation.

Elderly people are especially likely to develop arthritis, particularly osteoarthritis, which tends to affect weight-bearing joints such as the knees and hips. As a result, their activities are often restricted. They risk losing touch with their relatives and friends. Without companionship and the stimulus of getting out of the house, their discomfort and pain may become an overwhelming problem for them.

Although some elderly people live with their children, many live as couples or alone. Either arrangement may present difficulties for elderly people with arthritis and their families. Those who live with relatives and need extra care or help with personal needs may worry that they are overburdening those relatives.

"Meals on Wheels," "Friendly Visitor," and other home services are particularly valuable for older people. In addition, the elderly with arthritis need suitable recreational activity, which can be a wonderful stimulus and morale builder. Most communities have services of this kind. Golden Age clubs, day centers, and church programs offer organized activities and informal socializing for older people. These groups are sponsored by a variety of private and public agencies. If transportation to these activities is difficult, the centers themselves may have suggestions, or a neighbor may be willing to provide transportation in exchange for some other service.

In a few situations, an older person with arthritis may need to consider entering an extended-care facility. A decision about such a move should be made carefully, and only after fully exploring the possibilities and consequences. The change involves family separation, financial considerations, and, most important of all, the question of finding the right institution. Before reaching a final decision, the person thinking about such a move may want to discuss the idea thoroughly with a social worker in a family service agency or a member of the clergy.

Fortunately, most elderly people with arthritis can and do remain in their own homes, and do so with the cooperation of agencies in their communities that have been set up to help.

ARTHRITIS IN CHILDREN

Chronic illness in a child can be a heavy emotional burden for a family, troubling the feelings of everyone in the family. It is essential to sort out these feelings as the family deals with the disease.

Parents who are told that their child has chronic arthritis, one or both may react with numbness, shock, or disbelief. Other children in the family may feel rejected because of the amount of time and attention given to the ailing child. They may feel guilty, as if their normal sibling rivalry toward their ill brother or sister had somehow caused his or her illness. The parents may also feel guilty and ask themselves if something they did or didn't do caused their child to become ill. It is not unusual for one parent (usually the father) to reject the child's illness and to refuse to accept the seriousness of the child's condition.

The child with arthritis may experience a variety of emotions. Children can feel hurt by an illness that isn't their fault, blaming their parents for the illness, adopting a "why me?" attitude, and indulging in self pity or anger because of restrictions on their activities. They may also resent other children who are well, including their brothers and sisters.

The key to moving toward a healthy emotional climate in the family is open communication. Depending on the age and understanding of the child, the parents may want to communicate their own feelings to the child, which will encourage him or her to express his or her own feelings about being chronically ill. Parents may be surprised at how well adjusted the child is in dealing with the illness, but the child may also be angry at the parents for allowing painful tests, for not being able to stop the pain, or for limiting certain activities. Parents can help their child by allowing him or her to directly express anger from time to time.

In addition, parents may have to guide the behavior of other family members in relating to the ill child. Excessive sympathy or an attitude of ignoring the child's limitations are both out of place.

The relationship between the parents themselves and between the parents and the other children are sometimes set aside during the early days of a child's illness. Every effort should be made, however, to plan special times together and to communicate regret about any lack of attention the spouse or other children have received.

Parents should not be surprised that their own feelings and attitudes change as time progresses. Sometimes what originally may have seemed an impossible situation gradually becomes more tolerable as the disease is brought under control and the child improves. Most children with arthritis have long periods during which their disease is minimal and they can live nearly normal lives. During times when the disease flares up, it is important for everyone involved to maintain a positive and optimistic attitude yet at the same time to be realistic about the situation. Living with as normal a routine as possible will be beneficial to everyone in the family.

Most children with arthritis grow up to be adults without significant physical disability and flare-ups of disease become milder or cease altogether. It is important to make sure that they also reach adulthood without any emotional disability.

The child with arthritis may be physically smaller or slower to mature sexually than other children, may become easily fatigued, may have trouble keeping up with playmates and schoolmates, and may be unable to do some things other children can do. Without meaning to, children and adults often make matters worse by treating the child too gingerly. Special treatment can be upsetting, particularly during the teenage years, when being like other teenagers is important.

Some children with arthritis need encouragement to develop their potential capabilities. This need is particularly evident when they are in pain or are fearful about doing things that might hurt them. A child may sometimes use the illness as an excuse for not carrying out a job he or she dislikes. Angry feelings may emerge in refusals to take medications or to carry out a regular program of therapeutic exercise.

The attitude of parents has an important effect on how their children feel about themselves. It is only natural to try to protect a child with a disability, especially if the parents feel guilt or pity. But children will almost surely become dependent if their parents do everything for them or keep them from tasks they can manage themselves. If the parents do not expect much from their child, the child will not learn to feel useful and worthwhile. Children with arthritis must learn that they can do things and be successful despite their ailment. This will take time and patience, both for the parents and the child.

Parents can start building their child's confidence by not making special allowances, except for those that are clearly needed to avoid aggravating the child's physical condition.

They should expect the child to behave as well as other children, and to take part in family activities. This includes not excusing the child from light household chores, and setting limits for rebellious behavior. Being as consistent as possible will help the child learn what is expected.

Children with arthritis should also be encouraged to take active parts in their treatment programs. They should learn as much as they can about arthritis and about their treatment. The older child can and should be responsible for taking medications on time, reporting any medication side effects, and following the prescribed exercise program. The family must maintain control of inappropriate emotions and of times set for exercise, rest, visits to the doctor, and so forth.

Attending a regular school is also important for children with arthritis, unless they absolutely require special education. They should not be isolated from other children of their age. In fact, a federal law (Public Law 94-142) guarantees the right of disabled children to the same education as other children. This law stipulates that:

- No disabled child can be excluded from public education because of a disability.

- Disabled children are entitled to receive education and related services designed to meet their unique needs, including occupational and physical therapy, transportation, and vocational guidance.

- An individualized education plan (IEP) must be designed for each child. The parents are required to approve the IEP. If they do not agree with it, there are procedures they can use to change it.

In spite of the existence of this law, it is not completely carried out in every state or in every school district. If you have a problem in obtaining the services to which your child is entitled, contact the nearest chapter of the Arthritis Foundation for advice and assistance.

Teachers and school personnel usually want to be helpful, but also usually know little about juvenile arthritis. The parents should schedule a conference with the teacher and school nurse before the school year begins. During the conference, they should explain the disease and the child's treatment program. They should advise the school personnel that the child may have good days and bad days, and that morning stiffness may be a problem. This meeting is also the time to outline activity restrictions and explain any medications that the child must take during school hours.

The Arthritis Foundation chapters can help people find help in dealing with problems posed by juvenile arthritis. In particular, through the American Juvenile Arthritis Organization (a section of the Arthritis Foundation) families receive a regular newsletter with information relating to juvenile arthritis and the problems it poses.

Arthritis at any age is not easy to live with, but people who approach it realistically will find much they can do to modify, overcome, or rise above the problems it presents. People with arthritis need not face their problems alone. Physicians, nurses, other health professionals, family members, church members, public service agencies, the Arthritis Foundation, and countless others are available to help fill the gaps between what they can and cannot do for themselves.

WHERE TO TURN

Agencies	Where to look in the phone book
Arthritis Foundation local chapter	under Arthritis (if no listing, inquire of National Office; address in Chapter 26)
Community Council, or Council of Social Agencies, or Health and Welfare Council	under these names, and under the name of your town or county
American Association of Retired Persons	under this name
Vocational Rehabilitation, Department of	under the name of your state
Employment Services	under state listing

Agencies	Where to look in the phone book
Family Service Association of America, or other Family Service agency	under Family; or under the name of your religious affiliation; or call your Community Council
Legal Aid Society	under this name
Meals on Wheels	under Meals
Medical Society	under Medical
Mental Health Services	under community or county
National Council for Homemaker-Home Health Aide Services	under this name
Rehabilitation centers, independent Living Centers	under these names or under state listing
Social Security Administration	under U.S. Govt.
Visiting Nurses and Public Health Nurses	under Visiting; or under the name of your town or community; or under your city or county Health Dept.
Welfare Department (may be called Social Services in some communities)	under your city or county

CHAPTER NINE

Unproven Remedies and Diet Treatments for Arthritis

The use of unproven remedies or quack cures for arthritis is more widespread than most people realize. Approximately ninety percent of Americans with a significant degree of arthritis will try a worthless arthritis remedy at some time. It is estimated that people with arthritis spend more than one billion dollars each year on questionable treatments. Unproven remedies represent a tremendous drain not only on these people's pocketbooks, but also on their hopes and chances for successfully overcoming their disease.

What are unproven remedies? They are drugs, diets, or devices that have never been properly tested for their value in treating arthritis and are promoted to the public with extravagant claims, usually based on anecdotes. By contrast, legitimate experimental treatments are given only to carefully selected people with rheumatic disease, and only under the close supervision of physicians participating in strictly controlled, scientifically designed trials. The trials will reveal whether the treatments are beneficial and will help define how best to use them.

Part of the reason why so many people with arthritis break away from conventional treatment is their misunderstanding of the need for rigorous scientific study of all potential treatments for it. People who don't fully understand this need can be easily swayed by the claims of promoters of unstudied treatments.

Scientific studies are a crucial requirement before any medical treatment can be widely used. This is so because the results of well-designed studies are not clouded by large numbers of unknown factors. Outside influences are eliminated or are limited as much as possible. In a scientific study of a new drug treatment, for example, two groups of people with the same disease of almost the same severity receive exactly the same treatment procedures, except that one group gets the drug being tested and the other gets a placebo—a harmless, inactive substitute. Neither group knows which one gets the placebo. All other conditions, such as rest, exercise, other medicines, and pain-control measures, are the same for the two groups.

In this way, any statistical health differences between the two groups will be the result of the drug being tested and nothing else. If researchers notice that the test treatment works better than the placebo in preliminary studies, they conduct further tests to determine the safety, side effects, optimum dosages, and most appropriate uses of the treatment (that is, the diseases and kinds of patients for which it should be used). Other researchers will repeat the early experiments to prove whether the original results are consistent. All of these studies produce a backlog of evidence showing doctors how, when, and why to use a certain drug before it is marketed widely to the public.

Another important reason for requiring scientific studies of possible new treatment methods is that such studies take into account the placebo effect—the power of the mind in governing how the body will respond to a disease or treatment. People who want to recover and believe that they will recover when they try something new often do improve—temporarily. The placebo effect is not just a blanket term given to unexplained results; it has been shown scientifically to actually work; people often respond positively when given a harmless substance (placebo) instead of a real medicine. The placebo effect helps explain why some people respond well to treatments that are actually ineffective. In fact, testimonials in support of unproven remedies often come from people who were, in fact, benefiting from the placebo effect, or whose diseases just happened to go into remission at the time they tried the ineffective product.

Unfortunately, arthritis makes people particularly vulnerable to promises of easy solutions—for reasons related to the nature of the chronic rheumatic diseases. Arthritis and related diseases, for example, are often frustrating and difficult to live with. Most forms have no cure though they often improve spontaneously from time to time. Moreover, medical researchers don't know what causes most rheumatic diseases, but do know that most follow an unpredictable course of painful flare-ups separated by periods of remission. Persistent pain provides a strong motivation to try anything that offers the chance of relief. If a natural remission comes just after a person has tried one of the "miracle" products, that person is likely to believe that the product made the arthritis go away. Fortunately, physicians today know how to control many of the symptoms of the rheumatic diseases, while researchers continue to search for the causes and cures of this group of diseases.

People with arthritis want help. The best medical treatment is a far cry from the promises of the promoters of ineffective or unstudied treatments. The valid medical treatment of arthritis ordinarily involves a spectrum of activities that take discipline, time, and effort to follow. Doctors may stress that regular medication and exercise are needed to control pain and other symptoms, as well as rest, the use of helpful aids and devices, the pacing of daily activities, the use of hot and cold treatments, safe use of the joints, and, if necessary, surgery. The doctor will explain that improvement will come slowly and only if all aspects of the program are followed regularly. He or she will caution that some drugs don't work well for everyone, that drugs take time to become effective and may cause side effects, and that some people may need to try several medicines before finding the right one for their condition.

Many people don't like to hear such advice, and don't understand why their doctors cannot come up with a simpler and more effective program for treating their disease. They may feel that the doctor is giving them the runaround. Without easy access to the results of medical research, they lack an adequate understanding of their condition and of the latest treatment methods for it.

The promoters of unproven remedies have a far more enticing and visible message for people with arthritis. They offer either a cure or the quick, simple relief of pain. These people often claim that one remedy works for all forms of arthritis, and for other common conditions as well. As proof, they point to satisfied customers who tell of amazing improvements after using the unproven products.

The promoters of unproven remedies also call their remedies safe and painless, and condemn the medical profession's use of drugs and surgery as dangerous, damaging, and unnecessary.

Unlike scientific researchers, the promoters make these messages highly visible to the public in easy-to-read and sensational articles in tabloids and magazines. Many claim to have a "secret" or "exclusive" treatment, and charge or imply that the medical profession is a closed group that is slow to recognize and adopt real breakthroughs from outsiders. Many of these promoters also portray themselves as caring people who simply want to help others, and many claim to be victims of scorn and attack by the medical establishment.

Doctors dismiss the claims of these promoters, and explain that such "breakthroughs" would be unlikely to escape the notice of the hundreds of medical researchers studying the rheumatic diseases. They know that the products or remedies being touted have not passed rigorous scientific testing. Unfortunately, however, physicians often know little else about these products, since offbeat remedies are not usually described in the medical journals physicians read. The result is that when people ask their doctors about unproven treatments, many physicians can't readily give the reasons why such remedies are harmful or useless. Some people misinterpret this lack of familiarity as evidence that physicians don't have good reasons for their disapproval of certain unproven products.

Other influences besides testimonials and convincing advertisements also lead people to try unproven remedies. Often, well-meaning relatives or friends pressure the person with arthritis to try treatments of which they have heard or have themselves tried. Some people have difficulty refusing such appeals, and so eventually give in and try some offbeat treatment that seems to offer some chance for relief, however small. They hope that they may be lucky enough to hit on a useful treatment that medical researchers will explore successfully in the future. Unfortunately, their hope is misplaced; the legitimate willingness to experiment on themselves would have a much greater chance of success if they participated as subjects in properly conducted medical studies.

HARM OF TRYING UNPROVEN REMEDIES

Many people think that since the medical community doesn't know the cause or have a cure for most rheumatic diseases, they have nothing to lose by trying something promoted outside accepted medical practice. The truth is that while proper medical care does alleviate the symptoms and prevent or correct the deformities caused by arthritis, a few remedies can cause significant harm. Thus, some sources promote special diets that don't provide good nutrition, others recommend potent drugs that may cause serious side effects or interact dangerously with prescription drugs, and still others offer venoms, to which a few people are dangerously allergic. If you are thinking of trying such a remedy, contact the nearest Arthritis Foundation chapter to find out if it is harmful and if there is any likelihood it will help you.

On the other hand, some suggested remedies may be harmless, but may lead their taker either to delay getting proper medical care or to neglect his or her daily treatment routines while waiting to see if the remedy works. Meanwhile, serious joint damage can occur—damage that could have been prevented by staying with the proper treatment.

Unproven arthritis remedies are poor choices for other reasons as well. Such treatments waste money and—once their fraudulent nature becomes clear—can make the taker feel cheated, gullible, embarrassed, angry, and frustrated. Many people have reported having high hopes when they first heard the claims of some particular promoters, but that their hopes later sank into depression after the method failed to control their pain and other symptoms. People with chronic rheumatic diseases must already work very hard to overcome and resist depression. They should avoid creating more work and grief for themselves by pinning their hopes on false claims only to see their hopes of a cure dashed.

EXAMPLES OF UNPROVEN REMEDIES

Some of these remedies are easier to spot than others. They run the gamut from bizarre ideas, such as sitting in abandoned uranium mines to "soak up radioactivity," to approaches that sound impressively logical and scientific, such as elaborate procedures to "cleanse" the body of dangerous toxins that supposedly cause arthritis symptoms. Some remedies or clinics are even promoted by doctors, and can be difficult for people to distinguish from legitimate treatment.

Diet

Many unproven remedies are based on diet. Although good nutrition is important for everyone, especially people with health problems, no diet has been proved to prevent or cure any of the rheumatic diseases. Nor after hundreds of careful research studies, has diet ever been shown to make the symptoms better or worse in any form of arthritic disease except gout. People with gout do have to avoid certain foods that are rich in the natural chemical substances known as purines; these foods include liver, kidney, brains, peas, beans, and some others. They increase the uric acid levels in the blood and thus increase the chance of an attack of gout, which is caused by a buildup of uric acid crystals in a joint. Purines pose a problem only for people with gout, who have a defect in the way in which their bodies process uric acid (see Chapter 18).

Aside from gout, the most sensible advice about diet and arthritis is that people with this condition should eat balanced meals, and that those who are overweight should lose weight carefully. To have a balanced diet, a person must eat certain portions of food from each of the four major food groups every day. These four food groups are meats; vegetables and fruits; milk products; and breads and cereals. Together, they supply all of the nutrients the body needs. People unsure of their diets should ask their doctors or nutritionists for advice.

People who have arthritis and are overweight put added stress on their supportive joints, such as the hips and knees—a burden that should be avoided. Several studies have shown that osteoarthritis develops earlier and more often in people who are more than ten percent overweight. For such reasons, doctors often advise people with arthritis to help treat and perhaps prevent the condition by maintaining normal weight or by careful losing extra pounds. Any overweight person should consult with his or her physician before going on a reducing diet.

Using a common-sense approach to food is the best defense against the legions of special "arthritis diets" often promoted in clever books and magazine articles. The large number of different diet remedies is a strong clue that none really works. Some claim that avoiding the "nightshades" (the family of foods that includes white potatoes, tomatoes, and peppers) will clear up arthritis; others recommend taking high doses of certain vitamins; consuming food supplements such as cod-liver oil or extra minterals; avoiding meat and processed foods; or trying "allergy-elimination" diets. One person claims that different concentrations of homemade lemonade taken at very specified times of the day over a two-week period will cure arthritis. The list goes on and on.

Many scientists have looked carefully for links between diet and arthritis, particularly rheumatoid arthritis. Just about all of the studies have either no links or inconsistent ones at best. What have some of these studies revealed?

People with severe rheumatoid arthritis often do have nutritional abnormalities such as low levels of certain vitamins and minerals in their blood and tissues. These abnormalities are results rather than causes of the disease because the same abnormalities are found in other diseases characterized by chronic inflammation. It is also know that many people with advanced rheumatoid arthritis eat poorly, become run down, lose weight, and have anemia. When their disease improves as a result of treatment, however, they can overcome most of these abnormalities. Restoring their diets to normal usually helps these people feel better and improves their overall condition; but it does not affect the arthritis directly.

Peptic (stomach) ulcers and gastritis (inflammation of the stomach) appear to be more common in people with rheumatoid arthritis than in otherwise healthy people. This link, however, is probably the result of taking large amounts of aspirin and other anti-inflammatory drugs, and of the inflammation associated with rheumatoid arthritis.

On the basis of careful dietary histories, some people with rheumatoid arthritis have been found to consume calcium and vitamins at levels below the recommended daily allowances. When people without arthritis were examined for comparison, however, their patterns were much the same, thus making this finding only slightly significant.

Investigators have studied sulfur metabolism in people with arthritis, because this chemical element was commonly used in the past to treat many chronic illnesses, including arthritis. However, absorption and excretion of amino acids and other compounds containing sulfur are normal in rheumatoid arthritis, osteoarthritis, and ankylosing spondylitis. In one study, people with rheumatoid arthritis had low levels of one form of sulfur in the blood called sulfhydryl groups. However, similar low levels were found in kidney disease, certain cancers, and certain blood disorders as well.

Other scientists investigated the ways in which people with rheumatoid arthritis produce proteins. Almost all of the known amino acids—which are the molecules that serve as the building blocks of proteins—have been examined for abnormalities in people with this condition.

One group of scientists reported an abnormal breakdown product of the amino acid tyrosine in the urine of people with rheumatoid arthritis. This finding has been followed up by a number of other researchers, with inconsistent results. The particular abnormal material originally described has not always been found.

The blood concentration of an amino acid called histidine is sometimes abnormally low in people with active rheumatoid arthritis. To try to correct the low levels, dotcors gave supplemental histidine to these people and found that their bodies handled it normally. One study showed that the extra histidine had no effect on rheumatoid arthritis: the disease remained the same in people who were given histidine for eight months as in those not treated with this amino acid.

Many vitamin studies have been done on people with rheumatic disease. The nutritional status of some of these people has been poor, and vitamin deficiencies have been found. But while giving them the vitamins they lacked has cleared up the symptoms resulting from their vitamin deficiences, it has left their arthritis unchanged.

A defect in iron metabolism has been found in many people with rheumatoid arthritis. They do not incorporate iron normally into their red blood cells, which need it for the formation of hemoglobin, an oxygen-carrying protein. This defect is a common characteristic of the disease, but is not corrected by increasing the amount of iron in the diet.

People with rheumatoid arthritis may have osteopenia, the loss of bone substance. Because a major constituent of bone is calcium, scientists interested in the cause of osteopenia have examined how calcium is processed and stored in people with rheumatoid arthritis. Some studies suggest that these people don't absorb as much calcium from their food as healthy people do, but this difference is slight. A much more significant cause of osteopenia in people with serious rheumatoid arthritis is related to the use of corticosteroid drugs in treating this disease. These drugs are known to cause considerable loss of bone substance, particularly in women who have passed through menopause. Supplements of calcium and vitamin D in these people may reduce osteopenia but have no effect on their arthritis. Physical inactivity also contributes to bone loss, as do other unexplained causes.

Nutritionists and other scientists have also given considerable attention to the possible importance of trace metals—so called because they are normally present in tiny amounts in the body—in arthritis. They have been especially interested in copper, and have found that the amounts of this metal in the blood and joint fluid are higher in people who have rheumatoid arthritis than in normal people. Treatment with certain drugs, such as cortisone and penicillamine, lowers these elevated copper levels and brings about improvement of the arthritis. These researchers have concluded, however, that the elevated copper levels are a result of the disease, rather than a cause.

Another trace metal, zinc, has been studied in people with rheumatoid arthritis and has been found to be present in subnormal amounts. One investigator tested zinc supplements as a treatment for rheumatoid arthritis and found that at the end of three months, people taking the supplements were moderately better than those not taking them. The improvement was similar to that expected from the use of an anti-inflammatory drug such as aspirin in high doses. This finding has not been duplicated, however, and its significance is uncertain.

But even though scientific studies have not found conclusive evidence that diets of any kind help or cause arthritis, the dietary approach is still being widely touted. In fact, most bookstores carry several books that describe "miraculous" dietary treatments for arthritis. Somehow, seeing this kind of information in a book makes it seem legitimate to many people. They assume that the work would not be in print if it were false. Unfortunately, this notion is far from the truth. Because of our country's free speech laws, the writers of books can offer all kinds of medical advice; the consumer must take the responsibility to sort the good advice from the bad.

Some people promote diets that purposely do not contain certain foods, and claim that it is an allergy to these foods that causes arthritis. In these "elimination" diets, the person with arthritis is told to fast for a long time and then to add various foods, one at a time, to his or her diet to see if a certain food has an effect on the disease. This approach has been tried for arthritis since the 1930s, and is still being investigated. Although allergies cause a few forms of illness, research has not shown conclusively that arthritis is one of them. Occasionally, swelling in the joints occurs along with severe hives as a re-action to drugs such as penicillin or to insect bites, and may superficially resemble some chronic forms of arthritis. How-ever, this goes away when the body gets rid of the substance that has caused it. To date, no "elimination" diet has been scientifically shown to be of help for arthritis.

Venoms

Some unproven remedies use the venoms of ants, bees, or snakes as supposed arthritis cures. The direct danger in these remedies is that some people are highly allergic to such venoms —or may become allergic with their regular use—and can have serious reactions to them. A well-controlled study done in the early 1940s concluded that the slight degree of improve-ment noted in a few people with arthritis treated with a course of bee stings was not worth the significant drawbacks of this painful, expensive, and somewhat toxic form of therapy.

Plants and Herbs

Herbal or plant extract treatments are also touted as arthritis cures or remedies. They include preparations from alfalfa, the yucca plant, aloe vera, and Chinese herbs. Some people have promoted sea products including seaweed bracelets, mussel extracts, and even seawater as arthritis remedies. Part of their ploy is to use scientific-sounding reasoning to confuse people about mineral shortages causing arthritis.

Devices

Over the years, many ineffective devices have been sold for use in arthritis. They range from simple copper bracelets to intricate electrical or electromagnetic devices promoted for a variety of conditions. Some of these devices cause chairs and beds to vibrate, an action that may injure inflamed joints. Another device promoted in the 1950s and 1960s irrigated the colon with water and oxygen to flush out "toxins"; unfortu-nately, it also sometimes perforated the colon wall and caused serious infections. Radioactive devices such as mitts or bracelets containing crushed uranium have also been promoted for arthritis, but are useless, and give off little to no radiation anyway.

Lotions and Ointments

Some people with arthritis have rubbed on ointments, liniments, or special lotions trying to cure their disease. These products include DMSO (dimethyl sulfoxide), a controversial product that has received some scientific study but still has no proven effect on arthritis. A carefully controlled study of its use in scleroderma showed it was of no value in treating skin ulcers in that disease. Other such products are the mechanical lubricant WD-40 and weak mixtures of ingredients that give a slight warm or buzzing feeling to the area of application but do little else to reduce pain. Still other substances in this group include solvents and ointments containing salicylate, menthol, camphor, and numerous other ingredients (such as vitamins, special oils, or herbs); these preparations may produce some temporary pain relief by a counter-irritant effect. The active ingredients do not actually penetrate into the joints in therapeutic amounts as they are advertised to do.

Drugs

Some of the most dangerous remedies for arthritis offer false medication "discoveries" that are actually well-known drugs or combinations of drugs, herbs, alcohol, and acids. These potions may include hormone treatments (male and female hormones) or combinations of corticosteroid drugs, potent pain-killers, and illegal drugs such as cocaine. People pushing these "discoveries" often sell them in large quantities at high prices for use at home. They neglect to explain the dangerous side effects of using the medications over a long period, and they don't provide the close monitoring that such drugs require if used correctly. Some such drug treatments are sold from well-publicized clinics in other countries; others are sold in this country.

Miscellaneous Remedies

Many bizarre methods have been claimed to cure or help arthritis. Various claims include covering the body with cow manure twice each day; standing naked in the full moon; keeping two sesame seeds in the navel overnight while sleeping; and engaging in "foot reflexology" or unfamiliar versions of acupuncture to reduce arthritic pain. Acupuncture, when performed by trained health professionals, may reduce pain temporarily but can be expensive and probably produces most of its benefit through the placebo effect.

RECOGNIZING UNPROVEN REMEDIES

With all the treatment methods for arthritis that are promoted through newspapers, television, magazines, radio, books, friends, and relatives, how do you know whether any of them is justified or not? Before trying a new remedy or treatment, you should be cautious and suspicious, and investigate it. Many people with various professional degrees, including doctors, claim to have a cure for arthritis. But they often use telltale methods and gimmicks that help others spot them for who they are.

Here is a list of ten practices that are typical of promoters of quack and unproven remedies. Even if a doctor's name makes a claim sound legitimate, people with arthritis should be alert for these signs:

1. A cure is offered. There is no known cure yet for any form of chronic rheumatic disease. When genuine cures are found, there won't be any question about it; the whole world will know.

2. The cure or remedy is described as a "secret" formula or device—as "exclusive," or "special." Legitimate scientists don't keep their discoveries secret or exclusive.

3. Testimonials and case histories of people who have supposedly been helped by the remedy are offered as "proof" of its effectiveness.

4. The remedy or treatment is described in sensational articles in tabloids and special health-interest publications, or advertised in magazines and through mail-order promotions.

5. Quick, simple relief of pain is promised or implied.

6. The treatment is promoted as "cleansing" the body of poisons or "toxins" to allow the body's "natural" curative powers to clear up the disease.

7. Drugs and surgery are condemned as damaging, dangerous, and unnecessary. The person with arthritis is advised to try a nondrug treatment method.

8. No reliable evidence or scientific proof is offered to back up claims that the advertised remedy is safe and effective. The promoter has not had the method properly tested in clinical trials.

9. A special diet or nutrition treatment program is promoted as the answer to arthritis. Research scientists have not found any foods or nutrients that cause any rheumatic disease, or make any of these diseases better or worse (except modestly in gout).

10. The "medical establishment" is accused of conspiracy to thwart progress by refusing to "recognize" or "approve" the remedy being promoted. Particular targets include the Arthritis Foundation, the American Medical Association, and the Food and Drug Administration.

The best defense against unproven remedies is for people with rheumatic disease to take the responsibility for their own care, and to learn as much as they can about their disease. People who understand that symptoms come and go without warning and are aware of the placebo effect will not be conned easily by testimonials and "successful" case histories for an unproven product. Instead, they will learn about their disease from credible sources such as the Arthritis Foundation, community hospitals, or other reputable organizations. They will also report to the Arthritis Foundation when they encounter bizarre, unorthodox treatments, so that others can be alerted and educated to avoid these possible traps. The intelligent person will also ask his or her physician to explain the symptoms, treatments, and reasons behind any health advice that is given them.

With this knowledge, people with arthritis can become critical readers and listeners, and learn to ask questions and demand answers about possible remedies for the disease. Taking charge of their health care is their responsibility, and not that of their friends, relatives, or even doctors, who do not have to live with arthritis daily.

What can be done to protect the public against salesmen of worthless treatments for arthritis?

Three federal agencies are empowered to take action against promoters of ineffective remedies for arthritis or any other disease. The Food and Drug Administration can go to court to stop anyone from selling a drug for arthritis that has not been properly tested and approved for sale by that agency. The Federal Trade Commission can prohibit any individual or company from making false advertising claims for a product designed to treat any medical condition. Also, the United States Post Office can seize all mail addressed to any promoter who is selling such a product through the mail. Unfortunately, so many promoters sell worthless remedies that these agencies lack the staff needed to be fully effective in stopping these activities. In addition, many of these operators are careful to avoid breaking the letter of the law. There have been so many extravagantly advertised claims for DMSO, for example, that it can be sold successfully as "for use only as a solvent, not for any medical condition such as arthritis."

In addition to federal laws, some states have their own laws and enforcement agencies that protect the public from being victimized. However, many promoters of unproven remedies set themselves up so that they can make a quick profit on a given remedy before being put out of business. Then they quickly emerge with another treatment and so the cycle continues. An intelligent, well-informed public is the best defense against those who would cheat people with chronic illness by selling them worthless treatments.

Having responsibility, a positive attitude, and realistic hope will help you avoid the lure of the peddlers of unproven remedies. False hope is part of what such promoters sell, and their best customers are people without any hope of their own. As more people learn about rheumatic diseases, the promoters of unproven remedies will find fewer people willing to suffer the consequences of using their questionable treatments.

PART TWO

SIXTEEN FORMS
OF ARTHRITIS

CHAPTER TEN

Osteoarthritis

Osteoarthritis is a chronic disease of the joints involving breakdown of the joint tissue, primarily cartilage. It is perhaps the oldest and most common disease of humans and goes by a variety of other names, including degenerative joint disease, osteoarthrosis, arthrosis, and hypertrophic arthritis. Probably every person past age sixty has osteoarthritis to some degree, but only a minority has it badly enough to notice any symptoms. Sometimes, however, it becomes painful, limits motion, and requires medical care.

There are two categories of osteoarthritis: primary and secondary. Primary osteoarthritis appears without any obvious cause. Secondary osteoarthritis develops in joints that are known to have sustained damaging injuries. An example of secondary osteoarthritis is the condition called "baseball finger," in which a ball repeatedly hits a fingertip and the injury later leads to the development of osteoarthritis in that finger only. Secondary osteoarthritis may also occur in joints affected by infections, previous fractures, or by another type of arthritis such as rheumatoid arthritis. Sometimes, years of supporting extra weight (obesity) leads to secondary osteoarthritis in the weight-bearing joints.

AFFECTED POPULATION

Although anyone can develop osteoarthritis disease, older people are more likely than younger ones to develop it, possibly because of the buildup of joint damage from injuries and stress that occurs with time. When all ages are considered, women are affected about twice as often as men. Most likely, everyone who lives long enough will eventually get osteoarthritis to some degree, but most will never notice it.

An estimated seventeen million people in the United States have osteoarthritis seriously enough to cause pain. Because many more people may have it without symptoms, it is difficult to know how many actually do have the disease.

PHYSICAL EFFECTS

Osteoarthritis affects only the joints and surrounding tissues. In a healthy joint, the joint tissues are flexible and elastic, and movement is easy. In an osteoarthritic joint, the cartilage and other joint tissues break down, resulting in pain and difficulty of motion.

The first major change in a joint affected with osteoarthritis is that the smooth cartilage surface softens and becomes pitted and frayed. The cartilage loses its elasticity and is more easily damaged by stress. At first, the degraded cartilage cells are replaced, but this repair process eventually begins to fail. With time, large sections of cartilage may be worn away completely, leaving the ends of the bones unprotected. Without their normal gliding surfaces, the joint becomes painful to move.

As the cartilage continues to break down, the joint loses its normal shape and mechanical structure. The bone ends thicken due to growth of cartilage and bone and form "spurs" of bone called osteophytes at the points where the ligaments and joint capsule attach to the bone. The ligaments may also thicken. Fluid-filled sacs sometimes form in the bone near the joint, and bits of bone or cartilage called "joint mice" may float loosely in the joint space, contributing to the pain that occurs with movement. As a rule, only a moderate amount of inflammation occurs and is probably the result of loose pieces of bone and cartilage irritating the joint lining (synovium).

The progress of osteoarthritis varies significantly from one

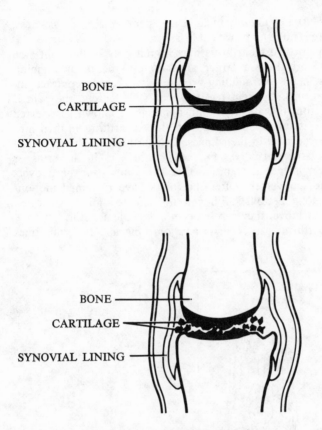

BONE

CARTILAGE

SYNOVIAL LINING

BONE

CARTILAGE

SYNOVIAL LINING

A normal vs. osteoarthritic joint

person to another. Some people have only mild changes that develop over a long period of time inside the joints. A few have joints that deteriorate quickly.

The symptoms of osteoarthritis also differ from one person to another. Most people don't feel anything before age forty unless they have injured or overused joints that are damaged or misaligned. When symptoms do occur they usually begin slowly and often seem unimportant. Most people feel a mild aching and soreness, especially when they move. Often, the symptoms do not progress beyond this mild stage. A few people have constant nagging pain even when they are at rest. Osteoarthritis usually doesn't include a general feeling of sickness, and there is no fever or weight loss.

The pain of osteoarthritis may be felt only in the joint area or may spread to a larger area around the involved joint. Muscles in the surrounding area may weaken or contract unnaturally, making them feel tense or stiff. Rarely, the pain is felt far from the affected joint, a sensation known as referred pain. For example, some people with osteoarthritis in their hips feel referred pain in their knees. Osteoarthritis of the spine can cause pressure on nerves that will cause pain in the arms or legs. Pain is felt most often after the joints have been overused and, conversely, after the joints have remained motionless for long periods. Although the affected joints are often difficult to move, they rarely become completely stiff.

Osteoarthritis can occur in any joint, but affects certain ones

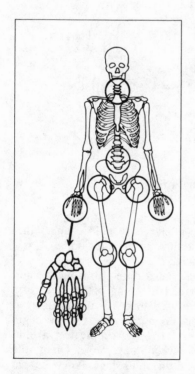

Joints commonly affected by osteoarthritis

more commonly than others. Often, it appears in one or a few joints and never involves others. The weight-bearing joints (those of the hips, knees, feet, and spine) are the joints most often involved. In the back, the bones of the neck and the lower back are most commonly affected. In the hands and feet, the finger joints closest to the fingertips, the joint at the base of the thumb, and the joint at the base of the big toe are among those that most often develop osteoarthritis. Other than as a result of injuries or unusual stress, osteoarthritis rarely affects the wrists, elbows, and ankles.

If the knees are involved, the major symptom is usually pain upon motion, which disappears with rest. The knees may feel stiff after the person has been sitting for a while, or when he or she first gets up in the morning. Sometimes there is a crunching sensation upon bending the knee. The area around the knee joint is usually tender, and sometimes the knee will catch or give way when it is moved.

Another type of osteoarthritis in the knee area is a softening of the cartilage of the kneecap known as chondromalacia patellae (the patella is the kneecap). This disorder frequently begins at age thirty or forty. Some people who have this problem also have a history of the kneecap slipping out of place. They have pain in the knee that is usually worse after unusual activity, especially after climbing stairs or taking long walks.

Osteoarthritis in the hip usually appears after age fifty-five, and may eventually involve both hips. This condition can become disabling. Its symptoms usually begin with a slow onset of pain followed by the development of a limp. The pain feels worse when the hip joint is moved, and is relieved when the joint is rested.

As mentioned, sometimes pain felt in the hip region is actually caused by osteoarthritis somewhere else, such as in the back. Hip pain that truly originates in the hip is usually felt at the groin or along the inside of the thigh. It may also be felt at the knee, where it may be so severe that the person experiencing it does not realize that it actually comes from the hip. This possibility is why doctors sometimes have the hips X-rayed in people who complain of knee pain. Pain may also be felt in the lower back as a result of the limp that develops.

Osteoarthritis in the bones of the back (the vertebrae) is common. It most often occurs in the joints of the neck and lower back, causing pain and stiffness in these areas. The cartilage between the vertebrae starts to wear away, and osteophytes form on the underlying bone. If these growths are located on the front of the vertebral bones they won't cause pain or other symptoms. If they are on the back of these bones, however, they may press on nerves, causing pain or even potential paralysis of the legs.

Osteoarthritis in the neck may cause shooting pain down the arms or up the back of the head; this "referred pain" is caused by pressure on certain nerve roots. Muscle spasm is another symptom of spinal osteoarthritis, and often leads to increased pain.

When the lower spine is involved, referred pain may shoot down the back of the thighs. This kind of pain is sometimes called sciatica because of the sciatic nerve, which carries pain fibers to the thighs.

Even though the pain of spinal osteoarthritis may be severe, serious nerve problems are unusual. The one exception is an unusual condition called cervical spondylosis, in which outgrowths of bone and cartilage on the vertebrae press on the spinal cord, causing weakness in the arms and legs.

A fairly common manifestation of osteoarthritis is the development of bony growths, or nodes, in the finger joints. Growths that occur in the end joints of the fingers are called Heberden's nodes, while growths in the middle joints of the fingers are called Bouchard's nodes. Either kind may result from an injury to a finger, but usually occur without any such event. They appear most often in women, usually starting between the ages of forty and sixty. They often run in families, which indicates an inherited tendency to develop them.

Heberden's or Bouchard's nodes usually appear first in one finger and may then develop in others. Some people notice sudden redness, swelling, tenderness, and aching in the affected joints, whereas in others the growths appear gradually, with little or no pain. The fingertips may feel numb and tingle, and the nodes make some people feel clumsy when they use their hands. Although the nodes may hurt, most people retain good use of their hands, and most who develop them never have serious problems in other joints.

POSSIBLE CAUSES

Although osteoarthritis has for many years been considered a result of normal wear and tear on the joints, this idea is now being questioned, and many researchers think that this disease can be caused by several specific factors. Genetics may be involved, especially considering the family link in nodal osteoarthritis of the hands. Some scientists believe that certain people develop osteoarthritis because they were born with defective cartilage. In a few people with rare, inherited defects of cartilage, osteoarthritis is more common than usual. Another theory is that some people are born with slight defects in the way their joints fit together or move; such defects may go unnoticed during youth, but after many years of using a joint, poor alignment may gradually wear down the joint tissues. Chondromalacia of the patella is probably such a condition.

Some people may develop osteoarthritis because a joint gets more punishment or stress than it can take. This punishment may come in the form of repeated, small injuries, the overuse of injured or badly connected joints, another kind of arthritis already present in the joint, or the joint having to support too much weight due to obesity. Athletes in certain sports appear to develop osteoarthritis more commonly, possibly because many fail to let an injured joint heal long enough before using it heavily again. Football players are more likely to have osteoarthritis of the knees, while baseball pitchers develop it in the shoulders and elbows. Professional dancers sometimes develop osteoarthritis in their ankles and feet, whereas these joints are rarely involved in other people. Pneumatic drill operators may find that their shoulders and elbows are affected. A study of many kinds of physical workers showed that the joints of the dominant hand (usually the right hand) were generally more likely to develop osteoarthritis.

Most scientists believe that osteoarthritis can also arise in people whose joints are aligned properly and have not been exposed to excessive stress. Considerable research is now being done to discover what initiates cartilage degeneration.

DIAGNOSIS

Doctors ask people suspected of having osteoarthritis to describe any physical stresses or injuries that may have aggravated or led to their pain. They may be able to diagnose osteo-arthritis on the basis of a person's medical history and physical examination, without the need for further tests. Sometimes, however, doctors do need special tests, especially when joints that usually don't develop osteoarthritis are involved or if many joints are affected, in order to be sure that some other rheumatic disease is not present.

X-rays can show the bone and joint changes that are typical of osteoarthritis. They may reveal whether there is narrowing of the space between the bones, whether osteophytes are present, or whether there have been alterations in the shape of the joint. The results of the X-rays do not always correspond directly with the person's symptoms. Early in the disease, the X-rays may be normal despite the presence of pain, since X-rays do not detect damage to cartilage, where osteoarthritis begins. More commonly, X-rays reveal definite osteoarthritis even though no symptoms are felt. Only about one-fourth of people with X-ray evidence of osteoarthritis have symptoms.

The physician may also order other tests to confirm the diagnosis or rule out similar diseases. He or she may draw fluid from the affected joint to see if infection or some other cause of arthritis such as crystals of uric acid is present. Another test sometimes used is the erythrocyte sedimentation rate, which may indicate whether or not inflammation is present. People with osteoarthritis only usually have a normal sedimentation rate. Other tests, including blood cell counts and the test for rheumatoid factor, may be ordered depending on the likelihood of some other form of arthritis being present.

TREATMENT

Treatment for osteoarthritis is aimed at controlling the pain it causes, improving and maintaining the movement in affected joints, and preventing or correcting joint deformities. It may involve some or all of the range of arthritis treatment components described in Section I: medication, rest, exercise, pain-control measures, joint protection, and sometimes surgery to repair or replace badly affected joints. The particular program depends on which joints are affected and how serious the symptoms are. The goal is to keep the symptoms under control, so that the disease interferes as little as possible with the person's activities.

The drug used most widely to treat osteoarthritis is aspirin. Aspirin reduces the pain caused by osteoarthritis and any joint inflammation that may be present. The other nonsteroidal anti-inflammatory drugs are often prescribed. Corticosteroids may be injected into osteoarthritic joints that have become inflamed. Other pain-relieving drugs such as acetominophen may be used for short periods during flare-ups of the disease but narcotics such as codeine are rarely used because people with chronic pain may become dependent on them. Occasionally, doctors prescribe muscle relaxants for people whose spine is affected and who have muscle spasms as a result.

The proper mix of rest and exercise is important for people with osteoarthritis. A joint that has developed degenerative changes can't tolerate the same stresses and strains as a normal, healthy joint. The person with osteoarthritis must learn the stress that his or her joints can take.

Particularly if weight-bearing joints such as the knees and hips are involved, avoiding their overuse is crucial. The physician may prescribe walking aids to spread the person's weight and spare the affected joints. Perhaps the most common aggravating factor in osteoarthritis of the hips and knees is obesity. The extra body weight puts a severe strain on these joints so that the disease is likely to become worse. Losing weight usually involves following a strict diet since people with osteoarthritis have limited exercise tolerance and use up fewer calories than people with normal joints.

For severe disease, the total replacement of joints with artificial ones often relieves pain and improves mobility. This technique has been one of the triumphs of modern surgery, and is particularly effective in treating advanced osteoarthritis of the hip and knee. In another type of operation, the bits of cartilage or bone that may be irritating an osteoarthritic joint are removed. This procedure may slow the development of further damage. Often this operation can be performed through an arthroscope inserted directly into the knee. Arthroscopic surgery usually requires a shorter period of hospitalization than regular surgery. Fusing damaged joints or cutting out sections of bone to improve alignment (osteotomy) to relieve pain is not done as often as in the past, but can be of value in some people.

THE FUTURE

The doctor follows the progress of osteoarthritis by periodically reviewing the person's symptoms and by examining the joints. In addition, X-rays may be taken at intervals to see if the joints are worsening. Since these changes usually occur slowly, such X-rays may be taken no more often than once every year, and usually less frequently. The physician will also review the effectiveness of the treatment program and make adjustments as necessary to maintain as much control of the disease as possible.

RESEARCH PROGRESS

Researchers are working on many different aspects of osteoarthritis, and have made promising progress. Until recently, most scientists believed that osteoarthritis was only a single type of disease that inevitably came from wear and tear on aging joints. Today they are realizing that it may have different causes and may not be an inevitable part of growing older.

Some of the research being done on osteoarthritis is focused on uncovering the differences between the cells of normal and osteoarthritic cartilage. Knowing this difference will help researchers devise ways of stopping the cartilage degeneration that occurs in the disease. Cartilage is made of two kinds of large molecules: collagen, a constituent of tough connective tissue, and proteoglycans, which are composed of proteins and sugars. The collagen forms a tightly woven framework into which the proteoglycan molecules are bound. The collagen in cartilage is somewhat different from the collagen found in the bones or the skin.

An important function of the proteoglycans is to trap water, and it is because of this ability to attract and hold water that normal cartilage can withstand pressure as well as it does. For example, when pressure is put on the knee by standing up, water is forced out of the cartilage as the surfaces flatten. When a person sits down, water flows back into the cartilage and its normal shape returns.

Research now being done on osteoarthritic cartilage is seeking the answers to several kinds of questions. For example, does something happen to the cartilage cells that are responsible for making proteoglycan molecules? Do these cells change in some way and start making defective proteoglycans? Or do the cells make proper proteoglycans, only to have some other substance attack and damage these proteoglycans? Is there a genetic component to the development of malfunctioning proteoglycans? Is there a genetic component to the development of malfunctioning proteoglycans? The answers to these questions should provide useful clues to the causes of osteoarthritis.

Investigators studying cartilage structure have found that osteoarthritic cartilage may have a defect in the "weave" of its framework. If this defect is serious, it affects the ability of the cartilage to bear weight. Normally the proteoglycans stick together to form large clusters. In osteoarthritis these clusters break apart. Researchers are trying to find out if prevention of this breakdown could prevent or slow the development of osteoarthritis.

Another possible explanation is that the proteoglycans in osteoarthritis do not retain water as efficiently as they should. Researchers are analyzing the proteoglycans in osteoarthritic cartilage and comparing them with those in normal cartilage in the hope of determining whether their chemical makeup is different. If any differences are pinpointed, the next step will be to learn how such differences originated. Another chemical approach is to study the proteins in joint fluid that are responsible for the lubrication of the cartilage surfaces as they rub against each other. A failure of the lubrication process might explain why osteoarthritis causes fraying, cracking, and erosion of the cartilage.

Medical researchers are also examining whether the collagen component of cartilage is abnormal in osteoarthritis. Collagen holds the proteoglycans in place and helps them attract water. If the collagen network is torn up, as may happen in a traumatic injury such as a football accident, the proteoglycans spill out like loose stuffing from a torn mattress. Sometimes, however, the collagen network comes unbound without any apparent cause. Some scientists believe that certain enzymes (chemical substances normally present in the body) may be responsible for breaking up the collagen network in such cases. In these studies, researchers must first discover whether the suspected enzymes are present in diseased tissue. One group of scientists is comparing measurements of enzymes in healthy tissue with those in osteoarthritic tissue to see if the enzymes in the latter are more destructive. They are also trying to pinpoint which enzymes, if any, are responsible for the destruction of cartilage. If enzymes are implicated, they hope eventually to design drugs that will stop these enzymes from going out of control.

Some researchers are investigating whether hormones are involved in osteoarthritis. Scientists became interested in this question because most women do not develop osteoarthritis until after menopause, when the levels of certain hormones decline. They reason that hormones such as estrogen may protect against the disease.

Some researchers are experimenting with ways of halting cartilage breakdown or of speeding up the body's natural attempts to repair cartilage. Others are investigating the differences between primary and secondary arthritis. These researchers are looking at how mechanical problems such as poor posture, flat feet, excessive weight, or injuries make people with these problems more likely to develop osteoarthritis. In particular, they are trying to find out why the kind of destruction that occurs in an apparently uninjured joint in primary osteoarthritis is the same as that which occurs in an injured or damaged joint in secondary osteoarthritis.

One of the most useful developments in the study of osteoarthritis has been the creation of animal models of the disease. Scientists have studied osteoarthritis in many different kinds of animals, but have been most successful with the rabbit. In fact, they have developed a strain of rabbit in which the disease—which may take years to develop in a human being—can be induced in a matter of weeks. By looking at the changes that take place in the rabbit cartilage, researchers have been able to describe in detail the different stages of the disease in the rabbit. This information is compared with information derived from samples of diseased cartilage taken from humans during surgery. If the rabbit model proves to be comparable to the human experience with osteoarthritis, it may be used to test ways of stopping the disease process in various stages of its development.

Some drugs thought to be useful in preventing osteoarthritis have already been tested in the rabbits in which the disease has been induced to develop. For example, research has shown that aspirin, although valuable in relieving the pain of osteoarthritis, has no effect on stopping the disease itself. The same is true of a drug called chloroquine, which researchers thought might prevent the breakdown of cartilage.

These and other studies are gradually clarifying the mysteries of osteoarthritis. As researchers uncover new information on the possible causes of the disease, its progression, and potential ways of slowing the cartilage breakdown that occurs in the disease, the goals of attaining better control and perhaps the prevention or cure of osteoarthritis become ever closer.

CHAPTER ELEVEN

Rheumatoid Arthritis

Rheumatoid arthritis is a common and puzzling illness. In its most serious form, it causes painful, badly damaged joints. But in its more frequent mild form, it causes discomfort but does not lead to serious joint deformity. Rheumatoid arthritis is a chronic disease that tends to flare up and subside periodically. It is systemic, meaning that it may affect many parts of the body. Although most people who develop rheumatoid arthritis improve on treatment and lead fairly normal lives, the disease is a major national health problem because it is a common, painful illness that can cause considerable damage to joints and disruption of the lives of those who have it. Rheumatoid arthritis is a major cause of economic loss in the United States every year. The basic principles of current treatment are somewhat better than those of ten or twenty years ago, and are being provided more expertly to more people than was formerly the case.

AFFECTED POPULATION

From one to three percent of the adult population—depending on how the diagnosis is made—has rheumatoid arthritis, which equals as many as seven million people in the United States. About three-fourths of these people are women. Although it can start at any age, the disease usually begins in midlife. Children also get rheumatoid arthritis (see Chapter 17).

PHYSICAL EFFECTS

The primary event is inflammation, which probably begins in the synovial membranes of the joints. It is usually most prominent and destructive at points where the synovial membrane meets the cartilage. A tongue of inflammatory cells, called a pannus, may form at that junction. With time, this continuing inflammation extends between the two cartilage surfaces of the joint and erodes the cartilage and eventually the underlying bone. Frequently, the supporting tissues, such as ligaments and

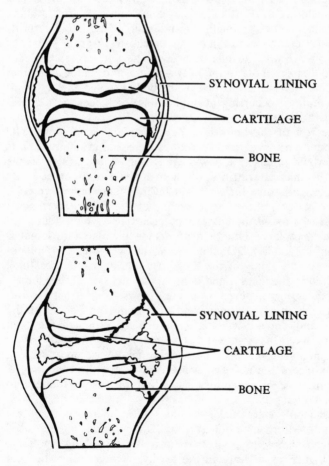

Normal joint vs. one with rheumatoid arthritis

127

tendons, weaken and the joints become unstable, dislocate, and become deformed, making all movement limited and painful.

The symptoms of rheumatoid arthritis differ widely from one person to the next, and often come and go without warning. Early in the disease, most people experience fatigue, soreness, stiffness, and aching. Muscle stiffness commonly occurs in the morning and after long periods of sitting or lying still. The stiffness usually eases after the person has been up and moving around for some time. A likely explanation is that fluid leaks out of damaged small blood vessels into the surrounding tissues during rest and then is pumped back into the bloodstream as movement occurs. Certain joints become warm, painful, swollen, and tender either gradually or suddenly. Rheumatoid arthritis typically affects several joints, unlike osteoarthritis, which is most often limited to one or a few. The joints most often involved first are those in the knees, hands, and feet. Commonly, the same joints on both sides of the body become affected, with the symptoms occurring in both hands, both feet, both shoulders, and so forth.

The rest of the body may be affected in many ways. The inflammation may spread to connective tissue in different parts of the body and cause a wide range of effects. Many people with rheumatoid arthritis lose their appetite and consequently some weight; some have a slight fever. Others may have cold, sweaty hands and feet or reddening of the palms. Swelling of the tissues around the ankles may occur. The lymph nodes and spleen can enlarge. Other effects include anemia (a low number of red blood cells), inflammation of the eyes, pleurisy (inflammation of the lining of the lung, resulting in painful breathing and fluid in the lungs), and lumps under the skin. These lumps, or nodules, often develop on the elbows, where there is frequent pressure; they come and go during the course of the illness and don't usually cause problems, although they can become infected. A rare but serious complication results from inflammation of the blood vessels throughout the body, leading to skin ulcers and nerve damage. Very rarely, this blood vessel inflammation, or vasculitis, can result in serious damage to internal organs and even death.

A person's emotional state may affect the severity of the symptoms of rheumatoid arthritis. Some people have noticed that their symptoms begin or return after disturbing emotional events, such as a death in the family, divorce, separation, or other emotional strain or shock. Physical injury to a joint,

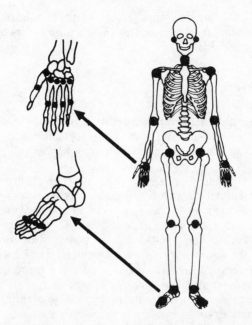

Common sites of rheumatoid arthritis involvement

such as a sprain or from overuse, frequently causes it to flare up. Most scientists believe that such events don't actually cause rheumatoid arthritis, but can often aggravate it. Even excessive worrying about having arthritis may delay improvement of the disease. When emotional and physical stresses are relieved, many people notice that their arthritis gets better.

POSSIBLE CAUSES

The cause or causes of rheumatoid arthritis are not yet known, but scientists have discovered some promising leads. As described in Chapter 2, many researchers suspect that a virus triggers the disease in people who have a genetic, or inherited, susceptibility to it. These scientists suggested that this virus triggers the inflammatory process of rheumatoid arthritis. The genetic susceptibility to the disease is associated with the presence of the human leukocyte antigen known as HLA-DR4 in the tissues of persons who have rheumatoid arthritis. Thus, while the HLA-DR4 antigen appears in about one-fourth of the general population, it is found in three-fourths of people with rheumatoid arthritis.

DIAGNOSIS

The diagnosis of rheumatoid arthritis is based on an overall pattern of symptoms and the results of a medical history, physical examination, laboratory tests, and X-rays, if necessary.

Several laboratory tests help the physician confirm a diagnosis of rheumatoid arthritis. Blood analysis usually includes the tests for rheumatoid factor (present in about eighty percent of people with rheumatoid arthritis) and for antinuclear antibodies (found in about one-fourth of people with rheumatoid arthritis), the erythrocyte sedimentation rate (which is usually higher than normal in this disease), and a red blood cell count (which is sometimes low—indicating anemia).

The doctor may also decide to include joint aspiration in his examination, so as to rule out the presence of gout, pseudo-gout, and infectious arthritis (described in later chapters). If rheumatoid arthritis has been present for more than a year, X-rays may be helpful in determining the degree of damage to the bones. X-rays taken early in the disease appear normal, but may be taken to provide a basis for comparison with X-rays taken subsequently.

Sometimes doctors order a bone scan, which is performed on a special type of X-ray machine. This type of scan can indicate the degree of inflammation in a joint, and may reveal early damage to the joint lining.

The physician may also do a biopsy of a rheumatoid nodule under the skin. Microscopic examination of a small amount of the material from such a nodule will indicate whether the nodule has the typical characteristics of a rheumatoid nodule or is caused by another disease such as gout.

The diagnosis of rheumatoid arthritis may not be made until after several visits to the physician. Because there is no one definitive test for this disease, the doctor may have to judge very carefully all of the available information, and observe how the individual is affected before making the diagnosis.

TREATMENT

Treatment for rheumatoid arthritis generally follows the basic plan already described in Chapters 4 through 6. Rest, exercise, pain-control methods, joint protection, and medication are all important parts of the program. Sometimes surgery (see Chapter 7) is also required. Of course, the specific treatment program for rheumatoid arthritis depends on the individual situation, because the disease can affect different people to varying degrees. The treatment depends on the severity of the disease, which joints are affected, the kinds of systemic symptoms that are present, and the age, occupation, and family situation of the person being treated.

The major goals in treating rheumatoid arthritis are to relieve pain, reduce inflammation, prevent damage to the joints, prevent deformities, and keep the joints movable and functioning properly. If the joints are already damaged, additional aims are to prevent further damage and to correct those deformities that have occurred.

In a few people, rheumatoid arthritis flares up to such an extent that hospitalization is necessary until the acute phase subsides. Most people, however, can carry on their treatment programs at home, with only periodic checkup visits to the clinic or doctor.

People with rheumatoid arthritis cannot expect dramatic overnight successes from treatment. Improvement comes slowly, and winning the battle against this disease takes great patience and confidence through its ups and downs and daily discouragements. Nevertheless, a proper treatment program, properly followed, will usually produce substantial improvement.

As described in Chapter 5, no single medication will cure or stop the progress of rheumatoid arthritis. Many different medications do help reduce the inflammation and other effects of the disease, and the doctor will try to find the best one for each person. Aspirin is the most widely used drug, but other nonsteroidal anti-inflammatory drugs are also commonly used for treating the disease. Corticosteroids taken by mouth are prescribed much less frequently—primarily for short periods during severe flare-ups. Injections of corticosteroids are sometimes given for temporary relief, especially when an extensive program of physical therapy or rehabilitation is being started. If necessary, the physician will recommend slow-acting so-called disease-modifying drugs such as gold injections, penicilla-mine, or antimalarial drugs for treating rheumatoid arthritis. The cytotoxic drugs such as methotrexate are used only if other medications have failed to control the symptoms well and the disease is severe.

Occasionally, drugs may also be necessary to treat the com-plications of rheumatoid arthritis. For example, a person may have to take antibiotics for an infection in a joint. Iron com-pounds may be given for iron-deficiency anemia, which de-velops in some people with rheumatoid arthritis.

A program including a balanced mixture of rest and exercise is especially important for people with rheumatoid arthritis. This program will vary, depending on how active the disease is at any given time. Attention to posture, the proper choice of shoes, and joint protection are also important.

Rheumatoid arthritis may produce emotional difficulty and depression. These effects are just as important to treat as the physical effects of the disease. Chapter 8 discusses strategies for living with a chronic form of arthritis that are particularly relevant for people with rheumatoid arthritis.

THE FUTURE

Although the course of rheumatoid arthritis varies from one person to the next, remissions of the disease may last for weeks, months, or years, even in people with severe rheumatoid ar-thritis. Furthermore, although a doctor may detect signs that the disease remains, the symptoms of rheumatoid arthritis eventually go away altogether in about one of every five people who have it, usually those who haven't had it very long. A small number of persons with rheumatoid arthritis—about one of every six—develop seriously deformed joints as a result. Fortunately, modern treatment methods can often minimize and delay the occurrence of these deformities and help correct them should they occur.

People with rheumatoid arthritis can take comfort in know-ing that medical researchers are making progress in under-standing their illness. Much of this progress is described in Chapter 2. As scientists learn more about how the cells of the body's immune system are involved in inflammation, they get closer to being able to stop chronic inflammation with new drugs designed to block the key steps in the inflammatory process.

Other researchers are exploring the connection between genetic markers such as HLA-DR4 and the triggering mechanisms that set off rheumatoid arthritis. Once these connections are better understood, physicians may be able to find ways to protect people who are at risk for developing the major forms of arthritis.

Important research on tissue changes inside joints affected with rheumatoid arthritis is also underway. Scientists have identified an enzyme called collagenase that appears in inflamed joints and is probably responsible at least in part for degrading the cartilage and other joint tissues. Currently, drug treatment for rheumatoid arthritis is aimed almost exclusively at controlling the inflammation in the disease, but joint destruction can occur even when the inflammation is under control. If scientists can develop a drug that keeps collagenase from harming cartilage, the joint destruction in rheumatoid arthritis may be at least partially preventable.

Research is also being done on a new technique called apheresis, or "blood-cleaning." This process removes specific cells from the blood, as well as proteins that are believed to contribute to rheumatoid symptoms. Blood is slowly and steadily withdrawn through an intravenous tube and processed so as to remove the harmful substances. The cleansed blood is then returned to the body through another intravenous tube.

To date, the results of apheresis therapy for rheumatoid arthritis are mixed; some people receive no benefit, others feel better for only a week or two; and some improve for a few months. At present, apheresis is very expensive and there is little evidence to show that it produces any lasting benefit to people with rheumatoid arthritis.

Although rheumatoid arthritis is a serious disease, the prospects are good for people who accept the challenge of overcoming its effects. Recent progress in the treatment of this disease has been significant, and the future appears even brighter.

CHAPTER TWELVE

Systemic Lupus Erythematosus

Most people have never heard of systemic lupus erythematosus, which is also called lupus, S.L.E., or systemic lupus. This disease, however, is not rare. It is an inflammatory disease of the connective tissues affecting many areas of the body in which such tissues are found. Although lupus is not primarily a form of arthritis, it is one of the rheumatic diseases, and its symptoms include joint pain and swelling. The disease may affect the skin, kidneys, nervous system, muscles, lungs, heart, and blood-forming organs as well as the joints. It is considered an autoimmune disease because the immune system produces an array of abnormal antibodies against human tissues that appear to cause some of the damage.

There are two forms of lupus: discoid and systemic. Discoid lupus affects only the skin. The word discoid means "shaped like a disc," and describes the patchy skin rash that is usually the only symptom of this form of the disease. This rash most commonly appears on the face, but frequently appears on other parts of the body. Rarely, discoid lupus may develop into systemic lupus. This chapter discusses only the systemic form of lupus because it is more severe and is the kind that frequently causes arthritis.

AFFECTED POPULATION

Lupus affects women about eight to ten times as often as men. Estimates are that several hundred thousand people in the United States have systemic lupus. It usually appears in women during their child-bearing years, although it can occur at any age in either sex. After the age of fifty or so, it is equally common in both sexes. For this reason, female hormones, which decrease after menopause, are suspected of being involved in the onset of lupus. Lupus also more often affects blacks and certain Indian tribes than people of other races.

PHYSICAL EFFECTS

Lupus may have remarkably diverse effects on the body; in fact, some scientists think that this disease may actually be a group of closely related diseases rather than a single one. The most noticeable effect of lupus is the production of abnormal antibodies called antinuclear antibodies, or ANA. These antibodies react against several chemicals in the nuclei of cells. A nucleus can be thought of as the nerve center of a cell, since it governs the activities of the cell—whether it will make insulin, develop into a red cell, produce cartilage, and so forth. The most important antinuclear antibody reacts with DNA, the material that forms the genes and thus determines all hereditary characteristics. This antibody is present in about eighty percent of people with systemic lupus when the disease is active. Other antibodies are directed against the red cells and cause anemia and some react with blood platelets, which are needed for blood clotting, resulting in an increased tendency to bleed. Research is still uncovering other kinds of abnormal antibodies in lupus.

In lupus, these abnormal antibodies combine with their antigens such as DNA and form immune complexes, which then circulate in the blood and deposit in tissues. The complexes are probably responsible for some of the tissue damage that occurs in lupus, since they collect in those areas of the body in which the disease becomes evident, such as the skin, kidneys, and joints.

There is no uniform pattern of symptoms in lupus. In fact, it may sometimes be difficult to distinguish this disease from rheumatoid arthritis. The disease appears in different forms and intensities, and varies at different times in the same person. It is often mild, but can become severe. Like other rheumatic diseases, the symptoms may come and go without apparent reason. Fever, weakness, unexplained weight loss, and particularly fatigue may be the first signs of illness. A rash may appear on the face, neck, or arms. This rash may be in the shape of a butterfly over the nose and cheeks. Most people with lupus become very sensitive to ultraviolet light, with the result that their rashes and sometimes other symptoms may appear or get worse after exposure to the sun.

Another early sign of lupus may be pain in the hands, wrists, elbows, knees, or ankles. This pain is the result of inflammation of the synovial membrane in these joints. Some joints may swell. The arthritis of lupus does not often produce the type of severe damage to bone and cartilage as found in rheumatoid arthritis. Not everyone with lupus develops arthritis. Other common symptoms of lupus include muscle aches, swollen glands (lymph nodes), lack of appetite, nausea, and vomiting.

Many people with lupus experience severe fatigue and depression, which may be a reaction to having the disease itself, to the changes in appearance caused by lupus, or to corticosteroids, which are sometimes used in treating lupus. Many people with lupus say they are often misunderstood by their friends and family members because they feel tired and run-down without showing obvious signs of illness. The person with lupus may be too fatigued to perform well at work or participate actively in family life. These effects may also contribute to the depression that affects some people with the disease. Counseling is often helpful in these situations.

As the disease progresses, some people with lupus may experience still other symptoms. It can affect the brain and nerves, impairing the ability to think straight or to remember events. Some people with lupus can actually become psychotic and have hallucinations or delusions. These episodes usually are only temporary. Convulsions, loss of consciousness, and even paralysis are other, rare events that can be produced by lupus. Additionally, the tissues that line certain parts of the body (e.g., the lung and heart) can become inflamed, causing chest pain. Kidney damage is often the most serious complication of lupus. For a long time this damage causes no symptoms, but as the waste products ordinarily excreted by the kidneys build up in the body, anemia, severe weakness, and loss of appetite result.

Only a few of these problems usually affect any one person who has lupus. Many people have only mild effects from the disease, and live happy lives without experiencing major health problems.

POSSIBLE CAUSES

Doctors and scientists don't know the cause of lupus, but research on this subject has provided many leads. Most scientists agree that something, possibly a virus, triggers the chain of events that lead to the abnormal autoimmune reaction in the disease. Some studies suggest that this triggering factor may combine with an inherited tendency to develop lupus, as described in Chapter 2.

Medical researchers have found that some medications taken for other conditions, such as high blood pressure, irregular heart rhythm, or tuberculosis, can cause a disease closely resembling lupus, referred to as drug-induced lupus. This condition usually goes away once the causative drug is discovered.

DIAGNOSIS

It's not hard to understand why lupus is often difficult to diagnose. It has many different possible symptoms and affects people in such different ways that a definitive diagnosis may require months or years of medical observation and many laboratory tests. A complete blood count is done to see if there are too few red cells, white cells, or platelets. A test for antinuclear antibodies will be performed, since almost everyone with systemic lupus has these antibodies in the blood. Other tests may be done to check for abnormally low quantities of complement in the blood, for antibodies against DNA and other components of nuclei, and to check the erythrocyte sedimentation rate (which is usually higher than normal).

Other useful tests include twenty-four-hour urine tests and kidney biopsies (to determine if kidney problems exist), chest X-rays (to see if the lungs are involved), and electrocardiograms (to detect any signs of heart involvement).

One of the first laboratory signs of lupus in some people with the disease are blood test results that are the same as those in syphilis. This result may, in fact, be mistakenly interpreted as a sign of syphilis rather than lupus. If the doctor suspects the result is false, he or she may repeat the test using another method. The second test will reveal whether syphilis is really present, or whether the results of the first test were actually an indication of lupus.

In a few people with lupus, the laboratory tests are normal despite other evidence of the disease. One problem in the diagnosis of lupus is that there is no single set of symptoms, pattern of the disease, or particular set of tests for all people who have it.

TREATMENT

Lupus is an erratic and unpredictable disease, and finding the right balance of treatment often takes time and trials of several different treatment methods. The treatment program for lupus ordinarily includes medications, exercise, resting when the disease is active, and being careful about sun exposure. It is important for people with lupus to let their doctors know when their symptoms change, so that their treatment program may be adjusted if necessary.

Because of the changing character of lupus, both the type and amount of the medications being used to treat someone with the disease may be altered frequently by the doctor. Some people don't have to take any medications, or must do so only when the disease is active. Sometimes aspirin or another non-steroidal anti-inflammatory drug is the only drug prescribed. Antimalarial drugs are also used successfully in treating active lupus particularly if extensive rash is present. Corticosteroids are often prescribed for people with severe disease, especially if the kidneys are affected. Sometimes, antimalarial and corticosteroid drugs are taken simultaneously. The use of corticosteroids has significantly improved the treatment results for people with serious lupus as compared with the situation of a few decades ago. Although doctors try to avoid the long-term use of these drugs whenever possible, the steroids are invaluable at times. If the disease has not improved after any of these medications, a person with lupus may be given cytotoxic drugs. Ointments or skin creams may be of some value in treating rashes. People with lupus who are sensitive to ultraviolet light should limit their exposure to the sun. Of course, what is too much for one person may be fine for someone else, but any person with lupus should take simple precautions, such as using a sunscreen lotion or sunblocking agent on their skin, and avoiding outdoor activities during peak sunlight hours. Many excellent sunscreens are available; those with a sun-protection factor of at least fifteen are generally the most suitable.

Because of the potential problem that sunlight represents, many people with lupus wonder if it is safe for them to move to a warmer climate. Lupus appears to be equally common in the south and the north, so by taking the proper precautions, people should find that their illnesses shouldn't be affected by where they live.

Adequate rest is essential for those with lupus, who often experience extreme fatigue. They need to avoid overactivity at work and at home, especially during flare-ups of the disease, and may have to consider getting household help or cutting back their work hours. Usually, they can continue with their normal activities, but have to reduce the time spent doing them. Such people may also need more sleep than other people do, and often benefit from short rest breaks during the day.

Certain chemicals such as hairsprays, paints, insecticides, and fertilizers have appeared to trigger lupus in some individuals, so anyone with the disease should wear gloves and protective clothing when coming in contact with these substances. Cosmetics should be used sparingly. Hypoallergenic brands are probably safest. Also, one should use temporary rinses or hair lighteners and take only drugs the doctor approves.

Some people with lupus can tell when a flare-up of the disease is coming on, and take appropriate precautions. The warning signals of a flare-up include general achiness, easy tiring, weakness, and a mild fever. These signs are an indication to call the doctor, who may recommend increased treatment measures to minimize the flare-up as much as possible.

Kidney Dialysis and Transplants

Some people with severe lupus develop serious kidney disease. If the kidneys fail in their job of removing waste products from the blood, techniques such as dialysis (in which a machine does the work of the kidneys) and kidney transplants may be necessary. Such treatments have saved the lives of many people with advanced, lupus-caused kidney disease.

PREGNANCY AND LUPUS

Women who have discoid lupus usually have no increased risk of problems with pregnancy. However, some of the drugs used in treating this form of lupus are suspected of being dangerous to the unborn child. Many doctors therefore recommend that women with discoid lupus stop taking these medications several months before conception and during pregnancy. The drugs should not be stopped before consulting the doctor.

Most women who have systemic lupus can have successful pregnancies, provided they do not have significant kidney or heart involvement. Although there may be hereditary factors in lupus, the disease does not appear to be passed directly from mother to her unborn child. The chances of carrying through a successful pregnancy with the delivery of a healthy baby are, however, somewhat less than in a person in perfect health. One of the antibodies sometimes present in the blood of women with lupus, called anti-SSA/RO, can cause damage to the fetal heart; thus, this antibody should be tested for in anyone considering pregnancy. Occasionally a woman who has lupus will have a flare-up during or just after her pregnancy. To be certain that pregnancy is advisable, a woman with lupus should discuss her situation with the doctor before she decides to become pregnant. If an unplanned pregnancy occurs, the doctor should be informed.

For women with lupus whose doctors advise them against pregnancy or who do not wish to have children, the safest method of contraception is the diaphragm used with contraceptive jelly. However, many women who have lupus use birth control pills safely; for them, oral contraceptives with a low dose of estrogen are preferable. Intrauterine devices (IUDs) are not advisable because of the high rate of infections connected with their use.

THE FUTURE

Most people with lupus do not develop serious joint deformities, and can lead full lives. They make the necessary adjustments during periods of disease activity, but otherwise largely carry on as they did before developing the disease. Lupus may come and go for months or years; in some people, it eventually goes away completely. Others experience repeated or changing episodes of the symptoms of lupus throughout their lives, but modern treatment usually keeps their health problems under good control. Most people with lupus need to continue to see their doctors regularly for repeat laboratory tests and physical examinations to assess how the disease is affecting them.

Recently, research has provided a much clearer understanding of what lupus is and better tests for diagnosing it, and particularly for defining the kinds of abnormal antibodies that may be present. Many improvements in the treatment of lupus have led to an increased life expectancy and an improved quality of life for most people with the disease.

Research on lupus erythematosus is a worldwide effort. Many scientists are studying the disease by using certain strains of mice that spontaneously develop diseases similar to human lupus. They can characterize many changes in the immune functions of these mice, and are comparing these changes with the findings in humans with lupus. These studies help to reveal the nature of the disease process, and allow scientists to test drugs that may appear promising against lupus.

Since lupus affects many more women than men, several studies have been done to see if the balance between female and male hormones has a role in susceptibility to the disease. Although the lupus that can be induced to develop in female mice can be alleviated by administering male hormones, this kind of treatment has not yet been applied in humans because of the danger of side effects.

Some researchers are investigating the use of prostaglandins —a group of chemical substances in the body with many different functions—in treating lupus. Certain kinds of prostaglandins may affect the kidney inflammation that is the fatal factor with lupus. Results from these studies could have a bearing on how humans with lupus-caused kidney problems are treated in the future.

Antiviral drugs are also being studied for use in treating lupus. Some scientists think that the disease may be triggered by a virus that lurks in the body for a long period before some set of circumstances activates it. This idea is supported by evidence that some antiviral drugs apparently reduce the kidney inflammation in some mice with lupus, thereby prolonging their lives.

Finally, the specific changes caused by lupus in the body's different kinds of immunologically active cells are being studied. These cells normally interact with each other in a carefully controlled, well-balanced system that governs our resistance to infection and harmful substances. Considerable evidence suggests that the factors that control this network of interacting cells go awry in lupus, with some cells becoming too active and others not active enough. Learning what these changes are and how to modify them may be critical in improving the understanding and treatment of lupus.

As research into lupus continues to reveal new findings, and these are incorporated into the treatment of the disease, the future outlook for people with lupus appears bright. No longer does this disease have to carry a frightening reputation; instead, it is being increasingly recognized as a disease that can often be controlled and overcome with proper medical care and the conscientious efforts of those who have it.

CHAPTER THIRTEEN

Scleroderma

Scleroderma, or progressive systemic sclerosis, is one of the lesser known rheumatic diseases. Like the others, it can affect people in different ways and to different degrees. Because scleroderma is a disease of the connective tissue, it may affect the skin, blood vessels, joints, and internal organs such as the kidneys, lungs, stomach, and bowel. The word scleroderma literally means "hard skin" and refers to the stiff and tight skin that most people with this disease develop over their fingers, face, and arms.

AFFECTED POPULATION

An estimated 50,000 people in the United States have scleroderma. Women are affected two to three times more often than men. The disease usually starts in the prime of life, between ages thirty and fifty, although it sometimes affects children and the elderly.

PHYSICAL EFFECTS

There are two kinds of scleroderma: localized or limited, and systemic or generalized. One form of localized scleroderma is called the CREST syndrome. Those affected by it have scleroderma predominantly in the skin and esophagus, and their

143

fingers are very sensitive to cold. The CREST syndrome and other forms of localized scleroderma may be disfiguring, but the general health of the person is only moderately affected. People who have localized scleroderma usually do not develop systemic scleroderma.

Systemic scleroderma can damage many organs. Besides damaging the connective tissue of the skin, muscles, and joints, it may also affect connective tissue and blood vessels in internal organs and structures. It can be mild or can occasionally become severe and widespread enough to be life threatening.

Connective tissue can be described as resembling sheets and strips of cloth, made up of "threads" of a fibrous protein called collagen. In scleroderma, the connective tissue cells make too much collagen, which collects in the skin and other body parts. These deposits of collagen cause the affected tissues to thicken and harden, and interfere with their normal function. Some researchers believe that a faulty immune system is involved in the collagen buildup because many abnormal auto-antibodies are present in the blood of most people with the disease. However, no one knows how the two events are related or whether one leads to the other.

An important feature of scleroderma is that the walls of the small blood vessels become inflamed and thickened, resulting in narrowing of the passageway for blood to flow through. The process may result from a buildup of collagen in the vessel walls. Scientists are unsure whether blood vessel changes are a result of the disease or a cause of the problems. Marked sensitivity to cold in the fingers as a result of abnormal blood vessels is usually the first symptom of scleroderma, so blood vessel damage is an early event in this disease. Ulcers on the fingers sometimes occur as a result of the narrowing of the small blood vessels.

Scientists have learned that the early damage to the blood vessels in scleroderma takes place in the vessel lining, called the endothelium. This lining consists of a thin layer of cells that lines the inner surface of the blood vessel itself and is in contact with the circulating blood. One of its functions is to keep the blood from clotting in the vessel. When the endothelium is damaged, the blood can leak out of the vessel, damaging the vessel wall and nearby connective tissue.

The first symptom of scleroderma is usually Raynaud's phenomenon, named after the man who first described it. It refers to an extreme sensitivity to cold that is most obvious in the fingers. The narrowing of blood vessels in the fingers and the resulting, greatly reduced blood supply cause the fingers to turn very pale in response to cold or emotional upset. Later they turn blue as fresh blood enters the hand but can't escape because of the constriction of the veins. Often tingling, numbness, or a cold sensation occur. When the hands warm up, the blood vessels eventually open and the skin color returns to normal as the blood supply to the fingers improves.

About ninety percent of people with systemic scleroderma have this reaction at one time or another, and sometimes all it takes to trigger it is walking into a cold room or reaching into a refrigerator. On the other hand, many people with Raynaud's phenomenon never develop systemic scleroderma.

Many researchers suspect that scleroderma is also an inflammatory disease, even though swelling, heat, or tenderness are not as evident as in rheumatoid arthritis. Although the joints themselves do not usually swell, most people with early scleroderma do have edema, or swelling, of tissue around the joints in the hands or feet, especially in the morning, for which reason this phase of the disease is called the edematous phase. When such swelling occurs, the skin appears shiny, the fingers swell like sausages, and the hands may be too puffy to close into a fist. A skin biopsy will reveal many inflammatory cells in the interior layers of the skin. These cells later disappear, and collagen begins to deposit. This sequence of events has led researchers to conclude that the inflammatory phase of scleroderma leads to the collagen deposits.

Sometimes, muscle weakness is an early symptom of scleroderma, and some people with the disease also develop small, white calcium deposits on their fingers. As time passes, ulcers or sores may develop on the tips of the fingers or toes. The skin on the face may eventually become tight, creating difficulty in opening the mouth wide. Chewing may also become difficult, causing trouble for people who use dentures.

Besides becoming tight and thicker, the skin may also become dry and coarse. The amount of hair on the skin usually decreases, and sweating may be impaired. Sometimes these changes occur only in the fingers, a condition called sclerodactyly. However, they may also occur in the hands, forearms, face, and other parts of the body.

Flexion contractures, or joints that tighten into a bent position, can develop in the hands and other parts of the body as a result of the tightening and hardening of the skin and tissues surrounding the joints. Flexion contractures can be postponed or prevented by range-of-motion exercises performed regularly every day.

Other signs may show up as the disease progresses. Small blood vessels in the fingers, forearms, face, lips, or tongue may dilate, or stretch, and become visible on the skin as the red, threadlike markings called telangiectasia.

Rarely, a person with scleroderma may not have any of the early symptoms or signs. The disease may affect only the connective tissue of the digestive system or some other internal body system, leaving the skin and joints untouched. If the digestive system is involved, the muscles in the esophagus (the tube that leads from the mouth to the stomach and through which food passes) may weaken and the lining become thickened by deposits of collagen. People with this symptom have trouble swallowing and getting food down the esophagus and into the stomach. A burning feeling in the back of the throat results from leakage of stomach juices into the esophagus. The bowel may also be affected by scleroderma, resulting in impaired digestion and severe constipation.

Other internal organs may also be damaged. The lungs are particularly apt to be affected, and serious difficulty in breathing may result. Kidney involvement can cause a serious and severe form of high blood pressure. Damage to the heart may cause irregularities of its rhythm and even heart failure.

POSSIBLE CAUSES

The cause of scleroderma is unknown. The disease is not contagious, nor is it inherited. Scleroderma appears to be an autoimmune disease. Scientists have found that in many people with scleroderma, lymphocytes have invaded the areas affected by the disease and stimulated the connective tissue cells to produce too much collagen. They suspect that some defect(s) in the immune system contributes to this lymphocyte invasion, but the agent that triggers this chain of events has not yet been found. Antibodies to nuclei are common, as in lupus, but they are directed against different nuclear materials than in lupus.

Recently, medical researchers have discovered an unexpected complication of bone-marrow transplantation that has shed further light on the connection between the immune system and scleroderma. Some long-term survivors of bone-marrow transplantation have developed skin changes and damage to their lungs, heart, and kidneys resembling the effects of scleroderma. The researchers postulate that the transplanted cells, which include cells that are precursors of immune cells, may react against the cells of their new host in a type of immune reaction. This finding also supports the theory that scleroderma is an autoimmune disease. A disease similar to scleroderma, however, can be produced by chemicals such as polyvinyl chloride, which affects mainly blood vessels. Certain drugs used in the treatment of cancer can cause effects in tissues that resemble scleroderma. Also, environmental factors may play an important role in producing this disease.

DIAGNOSIS

No single test or pattern of symptoms proves the presence of scleroderma. The diagnosis may take several office visits and perhaps some time in the hospital, and may include consultations with rheumatologists or dermatologists (skin specialists). As in any diagnostic process, the first step is a thorough medical history and a physical examination.

The tests done for suspected scleroderma may include a skin biopsy to reveal microscopic changes in the connective tissue. Another test that may be done involves checking the muscle pressure of the esophagus to detect digestive-system involvement. The esophagus may also be X-rayed. Blood tests may indicate imbalances in the relative quantities of different types of immune-system cells. The lungs may be examined and the breathing ability tested to see if they have become affected. Blood flow in the small vessels in the skin may be tested by subjecting the skin to temperature changes. Urine tests help the doctor determine whether the kidneys have become diseased. Using a magnifying glass, the physician also sometimes examines the small blood vessels in the nail beds to distinguish people with Raynaud's Syndrome from those with similar symptoms in the fingers who are developing scleroderma.

TREATMENT

The treatment program for scleroderma is designed on an individual basis, and takes into account the results of the physical examination and laboratory tests, the specific symptoms that exist, and the person's family and work situation. The program usually includes various medications, special exercises, skin care, and careful attention to meal planning if the digestive system is involved. The treatment may change as the course of the disease changes.

No "wonder drug" has been found to treat or cure scleroderma, but several medications are of some value. The doctor may prescribe a drug that causes the blood vessels to dilate, or enlarge, to treat Raynaud's phenomenon and the problems that come with it. These drugs include nifedipine (trade name Procardia), guanethidine (trade name Ismelin), methyldopa (Aldomet), and reserpine (Serpasil). Another drug sometimes used to treat Raynaud's phenomenon is phenoxybenzamine (Dibenzyline), a vasodilator that increases the blood flow to the skin and abdominal organs and lowers the blood pressure.

If the kidneys have been affected, drugs may be needed to control the high blood pressure that can result from this. Among the drugs used successfully to treat this complication are captopril (Capoten), propranolol (Inderal), clonidine (Catapres) and minoxidil (Loniten). Drugs that are used to control high blood pressure must be taken regularly, even when the person taking them feels well, because even though the condition may not always cause symptoms, it must be constantly controlled. The control of high blood pressure in scleroderma may be very difficult and require careful attention on the part of the person with scleroderma and the doctor to get the maximum benefit without side effects.

Some people show an improvement in kidney damage after being treated with drugs that control high blood pressure. Their skin symptoms may even improve. Since severe kidney disease may be life threatening in some people who have scleroderma, the possibility of reversing this process with medication is a welcome new development. In a few people with severe disease, drugs alone may not be enough to treat the kidney problems of scleroderma. Supportive measures may be required, including dialysis, in which a blood-filtering machine takes over the work of the kidneys.

Several drugs have been used for treating the skin problems of scleroderma, but physicians have no definite proof that they are beneficial. These drugs include vitamin E preparations, potassium para-aminobenzoate (Potaba), and the anti-gout drug colchicine. Dimethyl sulfoxide (DMSO) has been used extensively, but a recent controlled study showed it was of no value.

To prevent narrowing of the esophagus and heartburn, the doctor may recommend antacids, which can be purchased without a prescription. Cimetidine (Tagamet), a prescription drug that prevents the formation of stomach acid, is sometimes useful for this symptom.

If inflammation is present, aspirin or other nonsteroidal anti-inflammatory drugs may be given to the person with scleroderma. Steroids are rarely used to treat the disease, though some doctors feel that they may improve lung function. Recent research on other drugs, including penicillamine and immunosuppressive drugs, suggests that they may be used in treating serious scleroderma. However, these are toxic drugs that seem to require many months to produce any improvement.

Medication is only one part of the treatment for scleroderma. Many doctors recommend regular movement and exercise to help keep the skin flexible, reduce flexion contractures, and maintain better circulation. People who have scleroderma have

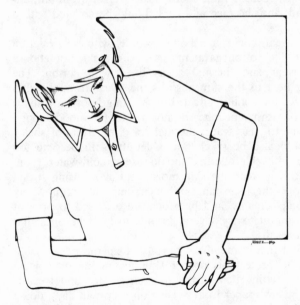

This hand-flattening exercise helps keep the skin flexible, reduces flexion contractures, and maintains better circulation.

a natural tendency to limit the motion of affected skin areas, and may need a greater-than-normal effort to move such areas. A daily exercise routine may be useful for such movement, and should be planned after consulting with the doctor or physical therapist. One useful exercise for the hands is to press each palm open on a flat surface at least once a day. People with joint involvement should also learn joint-protection measures (see Chapter 4).

Some doctors also suggest massaging the skin several times a day. Massage can combat the limitations of movement in scleroderma. A physical therapist can demonstrate the correct techniques for massage.

People with scleroderma need to keep their skin warm to avoid constriction of their blood vessels. During cold weather, they should always dress warmly to retain much of the body heat and help keep open the blood vessels to the arms, hands, legs, and feet. Wool garments are warmer than synthetic fabrics such as orlon, and wearing many thin layers keeps a person warmer than does one thick garment. Hats should be worn outdoors, since considerable body heat is lost from an uncovered head, and the face and ears should be covered with a scarf.

Because sweat cools the body, people with scleroderma should wear thin cotton garments next to the skin, or choose wool underwear and thermal socks lined with cotton. The cotton layer next to the skin absorbs the sweat from the skin and minimizes the cooling effect. Loose-fitting boots and shoes should also be worn, since they do not restrict the blood supply, and allow one to wear warm thermal socks or layers of socks.

Care should also be taken not to let the skin become too dry. People with scleroderma should use a cold-water room humidifier to help keep the skin moist, and avoid using strong detergents or other substances that irritate the skin. Many brands of soap, creams, and bath oils are designed to prevent dry skin; it is best to try several brands to find the ones that give the best results.

Friends and family members can also help the person with scleroderma to protect his or her skin, by taking over some tasks such as getting items from the refrigerator and freezer, picking up the newspaper from outside on very cold days, doing tasks involving putting the hands in cold water, and so forth. A person who lives alone and must take care of all household tasks can still avoid unnecessary cooling. Mittens or barbecue mitts can be worn when reaching into the refrigerator or freezer, and at the grocery store for handling frozen foods. A pair of tongs can be used to grasp ice cubes, which should be put in a thermal glass, so that cold beverages can be held comfortably.

Some people with scleroderma wonder if they should move to a warm climate. Although warm weather will not cure the disease, it may reduce the frequency of Raynaud's phenomenon and lower the risk of ulcers developing on the fingers. Many people with scleroderma feel better in a warm climate, but in most situations the slight improvement may not be enough to warrant taking on the expense and complications of relocating.

Doctors strongly advise people with scleroderma against smoking. In addition to all the other health reasons for not smoking, it may trigger attacks of Raynaud's phenomenon. Smoking causes the blood vessels to constrict, thus decreasing the blood flow to the fingertips. Smoking can also harm the lungs and heart, organs that are frequently damaged by scleroderma.

Another practice that seems to help some pleople with scleroderma and Raynaud's phenomenon is biofeedback training. This can teach a person to consciously increase the blood flow to his or her fingers and limit the blood vessel constriction that causes Raynaud's phenomenon. Since emotional stress also contributes to reducing blood flow, doctors often advise people with scleroderma to practice relaxation techniques and avoid stressful or tense situations if possible. Getting enough sleep is important for reducing tension, and counseling is helpful in learning to handle specific problems.

Doctors have several recommendations for people whose digestive systems are affected by scleroderma. Those who have trouble swallowing should eat slowly and chew thoroughly. Drinking water or some other beverage while eating will soften and wash down the food. Smaller meals are also a good idea; for example, eating six small meals a day may be easier than eating three large ones for someone having problems with chewing and swallowing. Another way to help prevent digestive problems is by not lying down for about four hours after eating a large meal. If possible, the largest meals should be eaten in the middle of the day rather than close to bedtime.

A further helpful suggestion is to raise the head of the bed

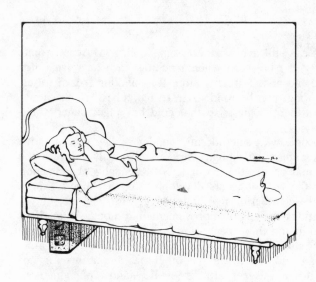

Raising the head of the bed will help prevent digestive problems that may accompany scleroderma.

by putting six-inch blocks under that end. In this way, gravity will help keep acid from backwashing from the stomach up into the esophagus during sleep.

THE FUTURE

Scleroderma remains a difficult disease to treat even though physicians understand much more about it than they did twenty years ago. Fortunately, in most people the disease remains limited to a few areas and progresses very slowly. In those whose disease is worsening more rapidly, there are often a few measures that are helpful in adjusting to the limitations imposed by scleroderma even though the process itself cannot be halted.

There are many techniques that the person with scleroderma can use to adapt to the disease. While most of these measures are not dramatically successful, they can make the difference between continuing a stable, well-adjusted and active life or becoming disabled by scleroderma. Most of what can be done to manage the disease depends on the person's own strong desire not to let it get the best of him or her, and on a common-sense approach to treatment.

Research on scleroderma is being done at many sites throughout the United States. Twenty years ago, very few medical scientists had any interest in scleroderma. A major national study describing the characteristics of the disease has recently been completed by the American Rheumatism Association section of the Arthritis Foundation. This study provides doctors with a much clearer understanding of what happens in scleroderma. The results of the study will help make earlier diagnosis possible.

Other researchers are studying the blood of people with scleroderma to see if something in the circulation affects the small blood vessels. The preliminary results of this research suggest the presence of a blood substance that appears to attack the endothelial cells that line the inside of the vessels. Whether this substance occurs only in people with scleroderma has not been determined finally. Another approach is to study connective tissue cells from people with scleroderma in tissue culture outside the body. Investigators have found that scleroderma cells in culture continue to make more collagen than normal cells. These results imply that either scleroderma cells have some genetic tendency to make more collagen or that they produce some factor that stimulates collagen production.

These studies and others like them also provide tools for researchers who are seeking the cause of scleroderma. In related research, scientists are trying to learn how to interfere with the mechanisms that are involved in the progress of scleroderma, with the hope of stopping the disease completely. Others are testing different drugs to find more effective ones for treating scleroderma. There is hope that in the near future more effective treatment and perhaps prevention may be found.

CHAPTER FOURTEEN

Polymyositis
and Dermatomyositis

Polymyositis and dermatomyositis are closely related, chronic diseases that affect connective tissues. In polymyositis, the primary process is an inflammation of muscles ("poly" means many, "myo" refers to muscle, and "itis" means inflammation), causing destruction of muscle fibers and weakness. In dermatomyositis, the muscles are affected by the same process but the skin is also involved ("derma" means skin). In this chapter, we will use the term myositis to refer to both.

AFFECTED POPULATION

Neither polymyositis nor dermatomyositis is common. In the United States, it is estimated that each year, five out of every one million people develop one of these two forms of myositis. Myositis can occur at any age, but most adults are affected between the ages of thirty and sixty and most children are affected at between five and fifteen years of age. Twice as many women are affected as men.

PHYSICAL EFFECTS

In myositis, inflammatory cells invade and damage the fibers that form the muscle tissue. The fibers break down and though some may be rebuilt, the affected muscles lose their structure and become weakened. The blood vessels supplying the muscles are also inflamed.

Myositis begins and progresses in many different ways. In most people, the symptoms appear slowly over a period of several months. In a few people, however, the illness appears suddenly. The symptoms may come and go for no apparent reason.

The major symptom of myositis is muscle weakness, with the muscles in the hip and shoulder areas the most commonly involved. The shoulder-area weakness often causes difficulty reaching up for objects or combing the hair. Hip-muscle weakness causes trouble getting out of a bathtub, bed, or chair, or climbing stairs. Other muscles sometimes affected are those in the front of the neck, making it difficult to raise the head when lying down. In severe myositis, other neck and throat muscles are affected, hindering the ability to swallow, and changing the quality of the voice. Some people develop weakness of the chest muscles and diaphragm, making breathing very difficult.

The person with dermatomyositis develops a patchy, reddish rash that may appear on the face, around the eyes, and on the knuckles, elbows, knees, or ankles. Some affected people also have puffy eyelids, frequently with a purplish discoloration on their eyelids.

Other symptoms of both polymyositis and dermatomyositis include fever, weight loss, and occasionally pain or tenderness in muscles and joints. A few people with polymyositis also have Raynaud's phenomenon, a reaction of the hands to cold (See page 144).

In about ten percent of adults with myositis tumors are found that may be somehow related to these diseases. Scientists have found that such tumors occur more often in people over the age of forty or fifty than in younger ones, and that children with myositis almost never develop the tumors. The tumors are more likely to occur in people with dermatomyositis than in those with polymyositis. The most common locations in which they occur are in the lungs, ovaries, breasts, and stomach, but they may also develop in or spread to other areas of the body. The key to successful treatment of these tumors is their early detection. Rarely, removal of the tumor results in improvement of the myositis.

POSSIBLE CAUSES

The cause of myositis is unknown, but because it appears in different forms, it probably has more than one cause. It may be an autoimmune disease, possibly one that is triggered by a virus in people with defective immune systems. Antibodies to materials in cell nuclei have been found in many people with myositis. These antibodies are different from similar antibodies found in systemic lupus and scleroderma. Myositis does not appear to be inherited.

DIAGNOSING POLYMYOSITIS AND DERMATOMYOSITIS

The diagnosis of myositis may require several office visits, perhaps hospitalization, and a range of tests. Though the diagnosis is usually not difficult to make once it is suspected, the weakness may be so mild a person may not complain of it and the doctor may not realize myositis is present. The condition resembles to some extent several other diseases of the muscles, and may appear in different forms from one person to another. The doctor may refer a person suspected of having myositis to a rheumatologist or to a neurologist, a physician who specializes in disorders of the nervous system, some of which may affect the muscles. Some individuals with rashes resulting from dermatomyositis may consult a dermatologist.

Several blood tests may be performed, particularly those for certain muscle enzymes. These enzymes are called transaminase, creatine phosphokinase, and aldolase. When a muscle is damaged, these enzymes spill out of the muscle fibers and into the blood. Tests that can measure the amount of these enzymes in the blood help the physician to diagnose and determine how serious the disease is. After treatment has begun, the doctor will repeat these tests to determine how well the treatment is working and whether the dosage or type of medication should be altered.

Other blood tests that may be done for diagnosing myositis include an erythrocyte sedimentation rate (which may be higher than normal), a complete blood count (usually normal), tests for antinuclear antibodies (present in about one-third of people with myositis), and tests for rheumatoid factor (which may or may not be present).

156

A very helpful diagnostic test usually used if myositis is suspected is the electromyogram (EMG), which measures the electrical pattern of the muscles. In myositis, this electrical pattern often shows characteristic abnormalities that help confirm the diagnosis.

The doctor who suspects myositis will usually perform a muscle biopsy to see if the characteristic picture of myositis is present. If myositis is present, the fibers usually show deterioration and signs of inflammation.

TREATMENT

The specific treatment for myositis usually includes medication, rest, and eventually exercise. It is usually effective unless the disease is particularly severe. Because the treatment is adjusted as the person improves, close cooperation with the doctor is important to ensure the success of the treatment program.

Medication is the cornerstone of treatment for myositis, and the most effective drugs are the corticosteroids. The corticosteroid most commonly used for myositis is prednisone. During the first phase of treatment, the doctor frequently prescribes high doses of this drug, perhaps sixty to eighty milligrams or more per day.

It is important to realize that it may take several weeks or months for improvement to become noticeable and for muscle strength to return. People in the first stages of treatment for myositis shouldn't become discouraged; they may be getting better without realizing it. Since large doses of corticosteroids may themselves produce weakness of the muscles, strength may not return until the inflammation has been controlled and the dose can be lowered. During this time and often throughout the treatment, the doctor may repeat the blood tests for muscle enzymes to watch for signs of progress.

After this first phase, the doctor will probably slowly reduce the prednisone dose to a maintenance level, which may remain the same for a long time. Depending on the course of the illness, the doctor may eventually be able to stop prescribing prednisone, at least for a while.

Some people, however, do not respond to prednisone therapy alone. The doctor may then prescribe both prednisone and a cytotoxic drug. Combining a steroid such as prednisone with a cytotoxic drug sometimes gives a good result when the steroid alone does not. Cytotoxic drugs interfere in some way with rapid cell proliferation, or overproduction. The inflammatory cells responsible for muscle destruction multiply rapidly and are very susceptible to the effects of these drugs. The drugs do, however, have serious possible side effects, as do the corticosteroids, which are described in Chapter 5. Anyone taking either or both of these medications should therefore become very familiar with the possible side effects, report any that occur, and keep in close touch with the physician.

In addition to medication, a physical therapy or exercise program is an important part of treating myositis, and can help improve muscle strength. Exercises or therapy should not be begun, however, until the drug treatment takes effect. In the early stages of treating myositis, the muscle fibers are still fragile, and can be further damaged by exercise and other forms of physical therapy. Physical examination and laboratory tests help the doctor determine the appropriate time to start an exercise program.

For this reason, people with myositis need to discuss with their doctors or physical therapists when to begin an exercise program and when to return to their usual daily activities. Returning to regular activities too soon may actually cause more harm than good.

Physical therapy for myositis can range from simple exercises done at home to formal sessions with a specially trained health professional. It may also include whirlpool baths, heat, gentle massage, or similar therapies. As improvement occurs, the program will be adjusted.

Rest is extremely important for people with myositis in the acute stage. During periods of increased muscle weakness, persons with the disease must take frequent rest periods during the day, and limit their activities. Fewer rest periods will be needed as the condition improves, but people with myositis should resist the temptation to increase significantly their activity levels at the first sign of improvement. On the other hand, complete inactivity may actually increase muscle weakness. The doctor or physical therapist can help decide the proper balance between rest and activity.

MYOSITIS IN CHILDREN

The outlook for children with myositis is generally good, although this disease may be quite severe in some children. Myositis in children is often a self-limiting disease, which means that the symptoms eventually go away after a single attack. The illness often ends as puberty begins, though it may disappear before this. Usually, it lasts only two years, although a few children may have a chronic myositis that lasts into adulthood.

In children with myositis, a condition called calcinosis may also develop, usually about two years or more after the myositis begins. (This can also happen in adults.) The presence of calcinosis indicates that the myositis itself is going away. In calcinosis, small lumps of calcium are deposited in the skin and in the muscle fibers. These deposits can be seen easily in X-rays of the affected areas. Sometimes calcium deposits near the surface of the skin break open and drain a white, chalky material. Calcinosis has nothing to do with how much milk or other foods containing calcium a child with myositis eats or drinks, so there is no reason to change the calcium intake of children with the disease.

Children who have myositis are also usually treated with prednisone. They receive smaller doses than adults, and don't have to take the drug as often. This treatment, combined with a physical therapy program, is usually successful in keeping the disease under control until it goes away.

THE FUTURE

Unless the disease is severe, the treatment of polymyositis and dermatomyositis usually works well. Although children with myositis may expect their symptoms to go away, adults are faced with a less certain outcome. For most, the prescribed treatment program usually brings improvement if the person follows it closely. Most people with myositis can lead essentially normal lives, although the condition may require changing some activities, especially during periods of increased pain and weakness. People with the disease may also have to continue taking medication and seeing their physician regularly. The disease is more serious if it affects the breathing muscles or is combined with a tumor; people with these complications will be monitored very closely by their doctors.

Researchers are making progress in understanding the physical effects of myositis and the changes that it causes in the muscles and in the body's immune system. Although the muscle fibers appear to be damaged by lymphocytes, there is a possibility that the damage is caused by abnormal antibodies. Recent studies have revealed a few kinds of antinuclear antibodies are more common in the blood of people with myositis than that of in healthy people. The results to date are not clear, however. In children most experts believe that the cause is an acute viral infection. Some recent studies have indicated that antibodies to coxsackie virus are more common in children with myositis than in those who have not had it.

As scientists get closer to understanding the process leading to the muscle damage in myositis, they can hope to find drugs that will stop the harmful effects of the disease. With the great progress that has been made in recent years, people with myositis have reason to be optimistic.

CHAPTER FIFTEEN

Ankylosing Spondylitis

Ankylosing spondylitis (also known simply as spondylitis) is a form of arthritis that primarily affects the spine, and leads to stiffness of the back. The term "ankylosing" means stiff or rigid, "spondyl" refers to the spine, and "itis" means inflammation. As a result of the inflammation in spondylitis, the bones of the spine, called vertebrae, fuse, or grow together.

In most people, spondylitis is mild and involves only the lower back. A few people have active, extensive spondylitis. With early diagnosis and proper treatment, the pain caused by this disease can be controlled, and serious deformity and disability minimized and perhaps prevented.

AFFECTED POPULATION

Spondylitis usually affects men between the ages of sixteen and thirty-five. Approximately 400,000 Americans are felt to have the disease. In women, spondylitis is generally limited in extent and is not often diagnosed. About five percent of people with spondylitis develop it in childhood. The disease occurs more rarely in blacks unless they have an admixture of white genes.

STRUCTURE OF THE BACK AND HIPS

Before learning some of the features and effects of ankylosing spondylitis, it is helpful to understand the structure of the back and hips, the two major sites of damage from the disease. The spine is made up of twenty-four bones, called vertebrae, which are stacked on top of one another from the pelvic bone all the way up to the base of the skull.

These vertebrae are separated from each other at joints, called the intervertebral joints, which allow the back to move in many directions. Within each intervertebral joint are discs that act as cushions, or shock absorbers. These discs are made of cartilage, which is softer and more elastic than bone and can expand and compress as the vertebrae move. In addition, there are two other sets of joints, called apophyseal joints, on the posterior part of each vertebra. As do typical joints, these joints contain synovial fluid, which helps them to move smoothly.

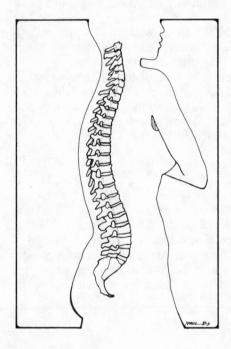

A normal spine

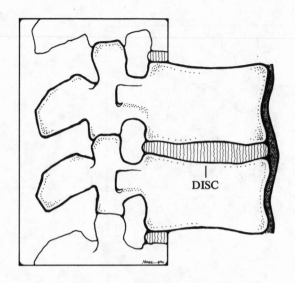

Normal vertebral anatomy

The spinal cord (the body's link to the brain) passes down the back through an opening in each vertebra. Many nerves branch out from the spinal cord, connecting it to the rest of the body.

The entire backbone structure is called the vertebral column. It is supported by strong muscles, ligaments, and tendons. It supports the upper body and allows it to move, and protects the spinal cord.

The lowest portion of the back is the tail bone, or sacrum. The sacrum joins the left and right pelvic (hip) bones, forming the sacroiliac joints.

PHYSICAL EFFECTS OF SPONDYLITIS

Spondylitis causes inflammation, which usually begins around the sacroiliac joints. Eventually, this chronic inflammation obliterates the cartilage that covers the ends of the affected bones, primarily in the sacroiliac joints and the vertebrae. The cartilage is gradually replaced by new bony growth, which ultimately fills in the joint space. This growth eventually forms a solid union between two neighboring bones, the condition referred to as

163

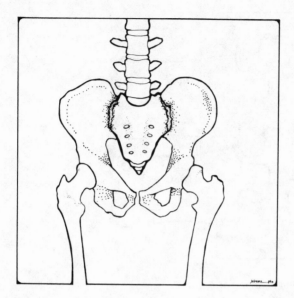

The sacroiliac joint

ankylosing. Why the result of inflammation in spondylitis (fusion of bone) is so different from that of rheumatoid arthritis (erosion and destruction of bone) remains an unsolved mystery.

Although spondylitis primarily affects the vertebral column and hips, other joints may also be involved. These include the shoulder, ribs, and, less commonly, the knees and ankles. Seldom are the hands and feet affected.

Sometimes spondylitis affects the ligaments that connect the ribs to the spine in back and to the breastbone, or sternum, at the front of the chest. The sternum may then become tender. Chest expansion is often limited by the fusion of these joints, although breathing is not severely affected because the diaphragm is not involved. The heels can also be affected by spondylitis, making it uncomfortable to stand on hard surfaces.

The most common early symptom of spondylitis is constant hip and low back pain and stiffness. Occasionally the first signs of pain and stiffness occur in the middle of the back or the neck. The back may become slightly rounded, and the chest may contract a bit. Left without treatment, the spine may begin to curve more obviously.

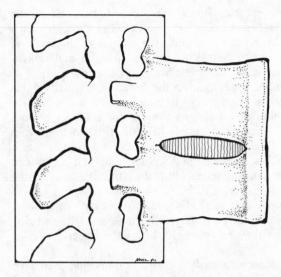

Vertebrae with the bony overgrowth of ankylosing spondylitis

Back pain caused by ankylosing spondylitis varies in intensity. Most people have only a mild ache in the lower back. The ache becomes more intense if a person tries to flex the spine by bending or reaching to the floor.

Some people with ankylosing spondylitis do not have back pain at first. Instead, their disease starts with pain and swelling of such joints as the hips, knees, or shoulders. This kind of beginning is most common for boys who develop spondylitis.

Back pain eventually occurs in almost everyone with this disease but it may not appear for a few months or even years after the other symptoms are noticed. In people whose disease develops in this way, the diagnosis is difficult to make at an early stage, unless other clues show up on X-rays, in laboratory tests, or during the physical examination.

Ankylosing spondylitis is a systemic disease and so may damage several different tissues. It may cause an eye disease called iritis, or anterior uveitis, in which inflammation of the outer chamber of the eye results in eye pain, redness, squinting, and increased tear production. Sometimes iritis occurs before the back pain or stiffness in spondylitis. Other systemic effects of spondylitis may include a mild fever, loss of appetite, weight

165

loss, fatigue, or anemia. Rarely the disease may affect the valves of the heart, particularly the aortic valve through which blood is ejected from the heart into the arteries of the body. If involvement is severe, corrective surgery may be undertaken. Lung involvement may also occur but is quite uncommon.

In early spondylitis, the pain in the lower back usually flares up and subsides intermittently. It may last for a few weeks, subside for a month or more, and return for a longer period. This pattern leads many people with spondylitis to think that they have merely strained their backs, and many don't seek medical help. A low backache and stiffness may first be noticed after some exertion or strain, but the stiffness and aching usually continues. It tends to be worst in the morning and to improve during the day, particularly after a hot bath or shower, or moving about. Back pain may also come at night and disrupt sleep. There may be referred pain in the upper thighs or knees.

Sometimes, people with early spondylitis think that they have a "slipped disc." Through a proper medical history, a physical examination, and sometimes X-rays, a doctor can tell whether a bulging disc is the cause of back pain in spondylitis.

As the disease progresses, the inflammation and pain usually decline as the affected joints continue to fuse. If the neck, back, and hips become fused in a bent or flexed position, a person's ability to do routine activities can be limited.

POSSIBLE CAUSES

Although the cause of spondylitis is unknown, scientists have discovered a strong genetic, or family, link. Almost all Caucasian people with spondylitis have the genetic marker known as HLA-B27 (see Chapter 2). Someone who has this genetic marker will not necessarily develop spondylitis, but people who do have it are more likely to develop the disease than those who do not.

Many scientists believe that spondylitis results from a combination of the HLA-B27 marker and a trigger of some sort, most likely some kind of infection. The trigger may set off a reaction by the immune system that becomes abnormal and leads to the damaging inflammation of spondylitis. Researchers are studying whether people who have the HLA-B27 marker have a defective immune system, which would lead to spondylitis.

There are several diseases that put people who develop them at a higher risk for getting spondylitis. These diseases include the inflammatory conditions of the bowel known as ulcerative colitis and regional enteritis (Crohn's disease), and the skin disease known as psoriasis. People with these diseases who have spondylitis are frequently carriers of the HLA-B27 marker, though some are not. However, even those who are not carriers have a higher risk of developing spondylitis than do people who do not have these associated diseases.

DIAGNOSIS

As with any diagnosis, the doctor will begin his examination for spondylitis by taking a medical history, seeking clues to explain the symptoms described. The physician will want to know whether other family members have similar complaints or have been diagnosed as having ankylosing spondylitis. During the physical examination, the doctor will pay close attention to the joints and other painful areas. Tenderness of the vertebral column and the ability of the column to move will be tested, and the ability to expand the chest is usually measured.

The laboratory tests done for spondylitis may include an erythrocyte sedimentation test to assess inflammation. A test for HLA-B27 can be performed but is expensive and seldom necessary to make the diagnosis. The doctor may order an electrocardiogram and chest X-rays to check for heart and lung involvement.

X-rays may also be taken of the sacroiliac and vertebral joints and of other joints that are suspected of being affected by the disease. Special bone-scanning techniques may be required if the X-rays do not provide enough information. To confirm the diagnosis of ankylosing spondylitis, the X-rays must show specific abnormalities. Often, however, changes do not show up on X-rays early in the disease.

Since most back pain is caused by conditions other than ankylosing spondylitis, physicians usually continue to examine anyone with unexplained chronic back pain, and may repeat X-rays of the back before making a diagnosis.

TREATMENT

The treatment for spondylitis is designed to reduce pain and stiffness, maintain flexibility of the spine, and minimize or delay curvature of the back. Each treatment program is designed individually, and some people improve more rapidly and steadily than others. The program takes into account the person's age, occupation, and usual activities, the severity of the disease, and its response to drugs. The ultimate responsibility for carrying out the program rests with the person involved, who really determines the degree of success that occurs. Even though the disease has no cure, treatment measures that are closely followed often help prevent major problems from developing.

Exercise

An important part of the treatment for ankylosing spondylitis is proper exercise. The doctor or physical therapist will probably suggest a program of exercises to be followed every day. The goal of such a program is to maintain good posture and strengthen the muscles surrounding the joints. For most people, following an exercise program every day will help maintain a posture and activity level that are as normal as possible.

For the person who sometimes feels too stiff and sore to exercise, a hot bath or shower will help loosen the muscles and joints. Exercises are most beneficial when begun slowly and planned for those times of the day when a person is least tired or has the least pain.

Exercises such as deep breathing will help keep the chest and rib cage flexible. Swimming or other exercises in water are also excellent ways to encourage deep breathing, strengthen muscles, and keep the joints flexible. One general goal of such exercises is to strengthen the extensor muscles, which stretch the body out, rather than the flexor muscles, which bend the body.

The doctor or physical therapist will explain how to do the exercises properly. They should be done every day and re-evaluated periodically with changes in the condition of the person doing them. The following are some examples of exercises that may be used to treat ankylosing spondylitis:

a) Spine-extension exercise. Lie on a bed on your stomach and stretch your arms out at shoulder level. Raise

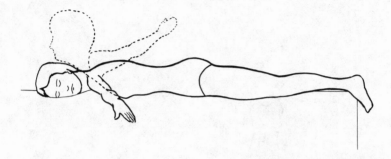

your head, chest, shoulders, and arms off the bed as far as possible. Then relax and repeat the exercise from ten to twenty times.

b) Chest-cage expansion. Lie on your back and clasp your hands behind your head. Pull your elbows down to the bed while breathing in deeply. Hold your breath for a count of ten, then exhale and relax. Repeat the exercise from ten to twenty times.

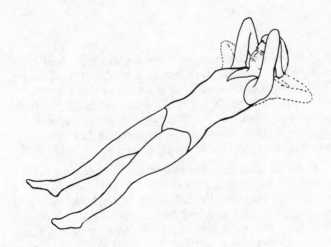

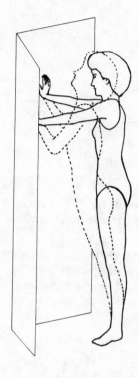

c) Combine the exercises for spine extension and chest expansion. Stand and face a corner of the room. Put one hand on each of two walls of the corner at shoulder height. Bend your elbows and lean forward. At the same time, extend your neck and breathe in as deeply as you can. Do this two or three times a day, and repeat it from ten to twenty times each session.

d) Other exercises. The individual exercise program for spondylitis depends on the exercises that are needed. There are special exercises for helping to stretch the calf and hamstring muscles and improve the function of the hips, shoulders, and other joints that may be involved. These may be prescribed if needed, as may additional back or chest exercises.

Many people with spondylitis wonder whether they must give up certain recreational exercises that they enjoy. Most don't have to, because their activities are beneficial in a general physical and emotional sense. Recreational exercises are excellent supplements to the specific therapeutic exercises for spondylitis that are prescribed by the doctor or physical therapist. Certain recreational activities and sports, however, are less suitable than others. For example, sports that require a lot of bending and mobility of the back are not recommended. Also, because people who have ankylosing spondylitis are vulnerable to injuries of the spine and neck, and have vertebrae that break more readily than normal, because the spine has lost its resiliency, they should not dive or engage in any activity that carries a danger of falling. Safe activities in which the back can be relatively upright are preferable. Ballroom dancing and fly fishing are two examples of safe, beneficial activities. The doctor or physical therapist can explain others.

Of course, activity must be balanced with the proper amount of rest, which helps control pain and inflammation. Short rest periods during the day help people with spondylitis reserve enough energy to get through the whole day without experiencing excess fatigue. The amount of rest needed depends on how active the disease is at the time.

Posture

Maintaining good posture is another aspect of treatment for spondylitis. A proper body position is important at all times—while sleeping, sitting, or standing—so that diseased joints will not fuse. Every effort must be made to keep the spine straight. Many doctors advise that people with spondylitis sleep on a hard mattress without pillows under the head, and sleep in a position that keeps the back as straight as possible, rather than in a curled position or with the legs propped up on pillows. Sleeping on the stomach will help prevent flexion deformities of the spine and hips.

It is also important to be aware of posture when lifting objects, walking, and sitting. People with spondylitis have to keep their backs as straight as possible and be sure that the chairs and work surfaces they use are designed so that they don't slump or stoop. For writing or reading, for example, a drafting table or upright stand may be preferable to a regular office desk.

Some people with spondylitis have limited joint mobility because a few of their joints have become fused. They may find it useful to talk to the doctor, nurse, or occupational therapist about the use of adaptive equipment and self-help aids. For instance, attaching long handles to such equipment as brooms or mops can help if the back or hips do not bend easily.

The Self-Help Manual for Patients with Arthritis, available through the Arthritis Foundation, includes descriptions of self-help aids and advice about posture and doing activities correctly to protect the joints.

Medication

While drugs do not cure spondylitis, they do relieve the pain and stiffness that it causes, thus allowing exercise to help prevent unnecessary deformities and disability. The drugs that are given may be changed from time to time as the symptoms of the disease flare up and subside.

Several drugs are used in treating spondylitis. For many people with the disease, the nonsteroidal anti-inflammatory drugs such as indomethacin are the most helpful drugs available. Although indomethacin is somewhat better absorbed when taken on an empty stomach, this practice may lead to stomach irritation, nausea, indigestion, and heartburn. If the drug is taken in the middle of a meal, it is less likely to cause irritation of the stomach. For many years phenylbutazone, another nonsteroidal anti-inflammatory drug, was widely used for the treatment of this disease. Although very effective, it produced a number of serious side effects, especially on blood cell production, so that most physicians try to avoid its use when possible.

Aspirin, which is often used in relieving the pain and inflammation of other forms of arthritis, has not been found to be as effective in treating spondylitis, although in large doses it can relieve pain and stiffness in some people. Corticosteroid drugs are also rarely used for this disease.

For the very few people in whom the heart is affected by spondylitis, digitalis may be prescribed to improve the pumping action of the heart, and other drugs called diuretics may be prescribed to reduce the amount of fluids stored in the body and ease the burden on the heart. People in whom the disease affects the heart usually require a low-salt diet.

Surgical Treatment

Improvements in the use of artificial joints are enabling some people with spondylitis to regain the use of joints that have been severely affected by the disease. The results of this type of surgery are more encouraging every year. Hip replacements are usually very successful and shoulder joint replacements are becoming increasingly successful. Some people whose backs are bent by fusion of the vertebral joints are helped by an operation in which a wedge of vertebrae are removed so the back is brought into a more upright position.

Other Treatment Measures

Because of the chance of lung involvement and reduced chest expansion, people with spondylitis are urged not to smoke.

Anyone experiencing eye problems should be examined by an ophthalmologist for signs of iritis, which can be serious if it is not treated.

SEXUALITY

Pain, limited motion, and other problems caused by spondylitis may interfere with sexual enjoyment, especially if the hips are involved. This situation does not mean that someone who has the disease cannot enjoy sexual relations, but rather that this may require some extra planning.

Many counselors advise people having such difficulties to think about what they do to make themselves more comfortable when lying in bed when they feel pain, and suggest that these same changes in position, especially lying on the side, be adapted to lovemaking, for the greater comfort and pleasure to both partners. Open discussions with the partner and health professionals can help the person with spondylitis learn to solve these problems.

THE FUTURE

People with spondylitis should expect to lead fairly normal lives. Most have mild or only moderately active disease. Despite the chronic nature of the disease, few who develop it suffer severe disability.

Often, the symptoms are slight and hardly noticeable. Ultimately, they may have little effect on the back and its movements. In a few people, symptoms may come and go over long periods, but eventually persist. The disease may leave permanent rigidity in the lower back and sometimes in the middle back, chest, or neck. Occasionally, other joints such as the hips also become stiff. Exercise therapy can help limit these effects.

Most people with spondylitis remain physically active and able to work despite their disease. If work must be stopped for a while during treatment of the disease, it can be taken up again after the inflammation has died down. Even those people for whom the end result of spondylitis is fairly extensive rigidity in the back are generally active and in good health, especially if the spine is not too bent.

Hardly anyone dies from this disease except from a spinal fracture, heart complication, or surgical accident. Even if the spine is severely involved, or if there is chronic arthritis of the hips or knees, the course of the disease is very slow. Routine activities are seriously affected only after many years of active spondylitis, and then only in a few people. The outlook, or prognosis, for most people who have ankylosing spondylitis is very good.

A major concern for people with this disease is that they lack normal flexibility and may fracture their spines after relatively minor injuries. They should avoid activities where injury is possible, like skiing, diving, or working on ladders or roofs.

Another cause for optimism is that researchers have made significant progress in understanding ankylosing spondylitis, and continue to add to their knowledge. For example, the study of genetic markers has provided doctors with important leads into how this kind of arthritis begins, and why certain people are more susceptible to it than others.

Researchers are also studying the link between certain infectious agents and ankylosing spondylitis. A series of agents, in a particular combination, may be responsible for starting the disease; the combination may be different for different people. The closer scientists get to uncovering the factors that trigger spondylitis, the more likely it is that they will be able to develop a form of prevention to protect susceptible people.

CHAPTER SIXTEEN

Reiter's Syndrome

Reiter's Syndrome, also called Reiter's Disease, is a form of arthritis that follows several kinds of infectious diseases. It is named after Dr. Hans Reiter, who described the major features of the syndrome in a German soldier who developed it after having dysentery during World War I. Along with arthritis, Reiter's Syndrome usually includes at least one of the following problems:

- Urethritis—an inflammation of the urethra (the small duct through which urine passes out of the body from the bladder). In men, this inflammation results in a discharge from the penis. In women, it may not cause any symptoms at all.

- Painless ulcers in the mouth.

- Conjunctivitis—an inflammation of the eyelids and the eyeball ("pinkeye").

- Keratodermie blennorrhagica—a chronic skin rash characterized by scaly, reddish patches that can occur on any part of the body, especially the penis.

Reiter's Syndrome occurs in people with a genetic tendency to develop the disease and is frequently triggered either by some sexually transmitted infections or by certain bowel infections. However, the microbes are not found in the joints; the inflammation seems to be a reaction to the triggering infection. In some people, the disease develops, remains for several months, and then goes away completely. Others have repeated episodes over a period of many years. The disease is usually not as serious as some other rheumatic diseases, such as rheumatoid arthritis, since it does not often produce permanent deformity.

AFFECTED POPULATION

Reiter's Syndrome primarily affects young men between the ages of twenty and forty, although it may affect anyone at any age. The disease is diagnosed in fewer women than men perhaps because its symptoms are very often not obvious in women.

PHYSICAL EFFECTS

Reiter's Syndrome begins with different symptoms in different people. These depend partly on what type of infection was present before the syndrome began. If the disease is preceded by a bowel infection, the early symptoms will include diarrhea, nausea, and vomiting. If it follows urethritis, the symptoms may be either mild or acute and obvious. In such a case the symptoms include pain or burning on urination and, in males, a discharge from the penis or urethra.

Several days or weeks after the symptoms of infection begin, pain occurs in one or more joints. The knees and the joints inside the balls of the feet are the most likely to be affected, but any joint may become painful. There may also be pain under the heels, in the lower back, and in the ribs. The affected joints are usually swollen and warm. Although the joints usually begin to improve after two or three weeks, many people continue to experience pain, especially in their backs and heels, even after their other symptoms have gone away.

Most people with Reiter's Syndrome develop the conjunctivitis with redness and irritation of their eyes. This complication usually appears during the first two weeks of a flare-up, if at all. It usually disappears of its own accord, without treatment, and leaves no permanent damage. Another symptom of Reiter's Syndrome is a type of skin rash that occurs in ten to thirty percent of people with the disease. It is a reddish rash that may appear on the soles of the feet, the palms, and other areas of the body. Usually, it is not painful or serious, and goes away in a few weeks. There may also be small red spots on the end of the penis, on the roof of the mouth, or on the tongue. Besides this, most people with Reiter's Syndrome have a slight fever, and some lose weight.

Some people have only a few of these symptoms and are said to have incomplete Reiter's Syndrome. For example, they may have arthritis alone, with no other features.

POSSIBLE CAUSES

The cause or causes of Reiter's Syndrome are unknown, but medical scientists have found some clues they are studying further. Most people who develop Reiter's Syndrome have had infections of their genitourinary system or enteritis, infection of the bowels. Why some people who develop these infections develop Reiter's Syndrome, whereas the majority do not, is probably related to a genetic susceptibility.

Genetic Markers

The HLA-B27 genetic marker, which is found in about eight percent of the general population, occurs in seventy percent or more of people with Reiter's Syndrome. It is the same genetic marker that is associated with an increased susceptibility to ankylosing spondylitis (see Chapter 15). Having the HLA-B27 marker does not necessarily mean that a person will get Reiter's Syndrome; it simply means he or she has a higher chance of developing it than do people without this marker. In fact, very few of all people with the HLA-B27 marker actually develop the Syndrome.

Infections

Although certain infections do seem to trigger Reiter's Syndrome, not all of the agents causing these infections have been identified. They are not found in the joints, which makes them more difficult to pinpoint as the culprits in the disease. Sometimes the disease seems to be triggered by certain bowel infections, particularly those due to certain species of bacteria, shigella, salmonella, and yersinia.

Scientists have been able to recognize that some of the microbes known to cause genitourinary infections can trigger Reiter's Syndrome in some people. They do know that such infections can be caused by several kinds of organism that are passed from one person to another by sexual contact; small microbes related to bacteria called chlamydia and ureaplasma have been linked to Reiter's Syndrome, but their role has not yet been fully understood.

DIAGNOSIS

The diagnosis of Reiter's Syndrome is based on the overall pattern of symptoms and on the results of a physical examination. The doctor will ask detailed questions about the joint pain and other symptoms a person is experiencing. During the physical examination, the doctor will pay close attention to the joints, eyes, and skin, and will look for other evidence of infection.

Although no blood or urine tests can prove whether or not a person has Reiter's Syndrome, such tests help to rule out similar diseases and to determine if an infection is present. The doctor may also remove some fluid from the affected joints to see if another kind of arthritis is present. Testing for HLA-B27 is sometimes helpful in making the diagnosis.

TREATMENT

Because there is no known cure for Reiter's Syndrome, treatment is aimed at controlling the inflammation caused by the disease and preventing or reducing joint damage. The goal is to keep the person with the disease comfortable so that he or she can continue normal activities.

The drugs most commonly used in treating Reiter's Syndrome are the nonsteroidal anti-inflammatory drugs. These help to reduce the pain and inflammation associated with the syndrome. Indomethacin is probably the drug used most often at first, although some other non steroidal anti-inflamatory drugs are probably equally effective. Although they can have side effects, as can all drugs, they often provide considerable relief in fairly low doses, so that side effects can be minimized or avoided.

For some people, a drug that did not seem to help at first may turn out to be effective several months later. For this reason, the doctor may need a trial period to find the best drug. In those few people who do not improve on treatment with non steroidal anti-inflamatory drugs, cytotoxic drugs such as methotrexate have been tried.

Mild skin rashes caused by Reiter's Syndrome are usually not treated with medication, since they are likely to go away on their own. Conjunctivitis may be treated with steroid drops if it does not disappear by itself.

Even though Reiter's Syndrome seems to be caused by infections, antibiotics have not proven to be predictably effective in treating it. This is because the microbes which caused the infections are not found at the sites of inflammation. Nonetheless, antibiotics are sometimes used, especially if the triggereny infection is known, in the hope that they will do some good.

Because of the close relationship between sexual activity and Reiter's Syndrome, doctors strongly recommend that men who have had this disease use a condom regularly, especially with a new sexual partner.

EMOTIONAL ASPECTS

Because of the probable connection of Reiter's Syndrome to sexual activity, some people who develop the syndrome are embarrassed by it. Some people even delay seeking treatment because they are hesitant about discussing their problems with a physician. Such people need not worry; the doctor will be concerned about the medical aspects of the disease, and will not judge their lifestyle.

Intimate personal relationships may also be harmed by Reiter's Syndrome. Communication between sexual partners will be awkward if either partner is embarrassed about discussing the condition. Part of this embarrassment may come from a changing body image. Such symptoms as a body rash or, in men, a discharge from the penis sometimes keep people from feeling good about their bodies. The person with a lowered self-image may well need some emotional support to restore his or her confidence. Patience and understanding are important ingredients in any couple's relationship, but may be even more important when one of the partners has Reiter's Syndrome.

Because no consistently effective treatment for Reiter's Syndrome has been found, some people may lose faith in their treatment and go "doctor-shopping" in an attempt to get well. But since each new doctor must start anew in seeking the best treatment for such people, the result is a loss of valuable time. People with Reiter's Syndrome need to understand their illness so that they will have realistic expectations of themselves and their physicians. The more they understand it, the better they can work with their physicians in finding the best treatment.

Some people who carry the HLA-B27 genetic marker are concerned about passing the tendency for Reiter's Syndrome on to their children. Genetic counseling may be helpful to those people who are considering having a family. However, it is very rare for two people in the same family to have the disease.

THE FUTURE

Some people have only a single episode of Reiter's Syndrome, after which the symptoms may disappear, never to return. Others may have repeated episodes with symptom-free periods in between. It is, however, fairly common for people with Reiter's Syndrome to have continuing problems, such as back pain or pain in the heels.

Researchers are getting closer to identifying the causes of this disease, with the hope of eventually developing effective prevention and treatment.

CHAPTER SEVENTEEN

Arthritis in Children

Arthritis is not just a problem of older people; according to some estimates, as many as 100,000 children in the United States may have some form of rheumatic disease. Children get several kinds of rheumatic disease, in addition to juvenile rheumatoid arthritis (JRA), among which are ankylosing spondylitis, lupus, and infectious arthritis. Because their parents have an important role in maintaining these children's physical and emotional well-being, they need to know as much as possible about their children's arthritis and its care.

This chapter discusses the forms of chronic childhood arthritis that are grouped under the heading of juvenile rheumatoid arthritis. Until recently, doctors thought that juvenile rheumatoid arthritis (also called juvenile chronic polyarthritis) was a single, chronic disease. Today, they recognize at least three forms of JRA, and have learned that the illness in children is different from that in adults. The prognosis for children with JRA is better than for adults with rheumatoid arthritis. Often, JRA involves only a few joints and lasts a short period of time, but it can also be serious. Its signs and symptoms can change from one day to the next, and even from morning to afternoon. Joint stiffness and pain may be mild one day and then so severe on the next that the child cannot move without great difficulty.

The parents of a child with JRA frequently feel discouraged because the disease seems to continue endlessly. Actually, most children do well in the long run. Permanent, arthritic damage to the joints is much less common in children than in adults.

Most children with JRA can keep up with school and social activities. Some changes will have to be made when the arthritis is particularly troublesome or if the joints have been damaged. By following the doctor's advice about medication and other treatments, however, most children with JRA can live nearly normal lives.

PHYSICAL EFFECTS

Each of the three forms of JRA begins in a different way and has different signs and symptoms. These forms are called:

- Systemic JRA, which affects many body areas, including internal organs

- Polyarticular JRA, which affects many joints ("poly" means several or many and "articular" refers to joint)

- Pauciarticular JRA, which affects only a few joints ("pauci" means few and "articular" refers to joint)

Inflammation is the major process that occurs in every kind of juvenile arthritis. The synovium that lines the joint becomes swollen and overgrown, and produces too much fluid. This causes stiffness, swelling, pain, warmth, and sometimes redness of the skin over the affected joint.

Because inflamed joints are usually painful to move, a child will often hold them still. However, lack of movement for long periods leads to stiffness of the joint and weakness of the muscles around it. Eventually, the structures around the joint may tighten up and shorten, producing the deformity known as a joint contracture. Doctors usually prescribe a physical activity program to help the child maintain a full range of motion of an inflamed joint and to keep the joint muscles strong.

In some children with severe JRA, especially the polyarticular form, long-lasting inflammation damages the joint surfaces. This process can result in the kinds of deformity many people have seen in adults with rheumatoid arthritis. Fortunately, this extreme result is rare.

Sometimes joint inflammation speeds up or slows down the growth centers in bones. The affected bones may become longer or shorter than normal. When long-standing arthritis affects the growth centers of many bones, a child's general physical development may be slowed. Growth usually resumes when the disease is brought under control, although a child who has had JRA may not grow to previously expected height.

Although inflammation is common to all three forms of JRA, they differ in the specific joint problems and other symptoms they cause. These differences are described in the following section.

Systemic Juvenile Rheumatoid Arthritis

The term Still's disease is often used to refer to this form, since it was originally described by Dr. G. F. Still in 1897. Boys and girls are equally likely to get this kind of JRA. It affects children of any age, and is responsible for about twenty percent of all cases of JRA.

High fevers are a frequent symptom of systemic JRA. The fever usually starts in the evening. The child's temperature generally goes up to 103 degrees or higher, and then comes back down to normal within a few hours, only to rise again the next day. Shaking chills often accompany the fever, and the child may feel very sick. Periods of fever can last for weeks or even months, but rarely go on for more than six months.

Children with systemic JRA also often develop a characteristic rash when they have a fever. This rash comes and goes for many days in a row. It may be present only briefly, when the temperature is up. Pale red spots often appear on the child's chest and thighs and sometimes on other parts of the body. They may come on after a hot tub bath or shower. The parent should look for this rash because its presence is very helpful to the physician in making a diagnosis. Often it is absent when the physician happens to examine the child.

The arthritis of systemic JRA generally affects many joints. The joint problems may begin with the fever or start weeks or months later. Some children have severe pain in their joints when they have a fever and then feel much better when their temperature goes down. Joint problems may also continue after the fever period ends, and may be a major long-term difficulty for children with systemic JRA.

Other effects of systemic JRA may be inflammation of the outer lining of the heart (pericarditis) or the lungs (pleuritis), stomach pain, severe anemia, and a high number of white cells in the blood. Regular visits to the doctor are important so that these effects can be monitored and treated from the beginning. When the disease is severe the child may be extremely ill and need to enter the hospital.

Polyarticular Juvenile Rheumatoid Arthritis

It is estimated that forty to fifty percent of all children with JRA have the polyarticular form. Girls develop polyarticular arthritis more often than boys.

Polyarticular JRA appears in five or more joints, usually including the small joints of the fingers and hands, and sometimes the weight-bearing joints (hips, knees, ankles, and feet). The disease is often symmetrical, meaning that the same joint on both sides of the body is involved. Some children also have slight fevers.

Some children with polyarticular JRA have rheumatoid

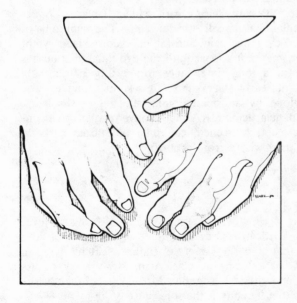

Symmetrical joint involvement in polyarticular JRA

factor in their blood. They are most likely to develop rheumatoid nodules on their elbows or other points of the body that receive pressure from chairs, shoes, and other sources. They also have more of a tendency to have long-lasting disease extending into adulthood. Their disease seems to be identical to adult rheumatoid arthritis.

Pauciarticular Juvenile Rheumatoid Arthritis

Children with pauciarticular JRA account for thirty to forty percent of all those with JRA. This type of JRA affects only a few joints (four or less), usually large joints such as the knees, ankles, or elbows. It seldom affects the same joint on both sides of the body. There are two subtypes of pauciarticular JRA, one that develops primarily in boys and the other primarily in girls.

Some boys with pauciarticular JRA are likely to have stiffness in the hips and lower back early in the disease, in addition to arthritis in the large joints. They often later develop the adult form of arthritis called ankylosing spondylitis, which affects the spine and hips (see Chapter 16).

Some children (usually girls) with pauciarticular JRA develop an eye inflammation called iridocyclitis. The symptoms of this include red eyes, eye pain, and failing vision. These symptoms, however, may not appear until the eye inflammation has been present for a long time. Since iridocyclitis can usually be detected in its early stages, through a simple, painless eye examination done by an ophthalmologist using a slit lamp, children with pauciarticular JRA should have regular eye examinations. Treatment, if needed, can then be started early to prevent any loss of vision from occurring.

POSSIBLE CAUSES

Scientists don't know what causes any of the forms of juvenile rheumatoid arthritis. They do know that JRA is not contagious, and that a child therefore cannot "catch" it from anyone or give it to someone else. Also, JRA rarely occurs in more than one child in a family, for which reason doctors do not believe that heredity is the sole cause of any type.

186

Considerable research is underway to find the cause or causes of JRA.

DIAGNOSIS

Because the signs and symptoms of JRA can vary so much from one child to another, diagnosis can be difficult. Many steps may be involved in finding out if a child really does have JRA, and if so, what type. The major steps are the medical history, a physical examination, laboratory tests, and an X-ray examination. Sometimes samples of joint fluid or tissue will also be examined.

The doctor will question the child and parents about how the child has been feeling recently and what has happened during his or her lifetime and during the present illness that may affect the disease. The doctor will also find out how long the symptoms have been present and try to uncover how they began. Many infections caused by viruses can lead to arthritis in children, but in these situations the arthritis usually goes away rapidly. To make a diagnosis of chronic JRA, the arthritis must have been present for six or more consecutive weeks. Some children, especially very young ones, seem to have a diminished awareness of pain. Such a child may not complain of joint pain when arthritis is present. The parent may notice that the child has a slight limp or is reluctant to be as physically active in games or other activities before he or she became affected.

The doctor may also want to know if other members of the family have had arthritis, particularly ankylosing spondylitis, since this type of arthritis may be inherited.

The doctor will do a physical examination, paying special attention to the child's joints. The doctor must be able to find evidence of joint inflammation to be sure that JRA is the problem. A child who complains of aches and pains but who shows no joint changes may not have JRA. In the systemic form, however, joint involvement may not be detectable early in the disease.

The doctor will also look for other signs of JRA, such as the rash that goes with systemic JRA or the nodules that can be present in polyarticular JRA. If there is any possibility of eye involvement, the child will be sent to an ophthalmologist for a slit lamp examination. This test should be repeated from time to time in any child with JRA.

Several laboratory tests can help the doctor decide whether a child has JRA, and which type of JRA it is. No single test provides proof that the disease is present or not. Diagnostic blood tests may include the erythrocyte sedimentation rate, rheumatoid factor test, antinuclear antibody test, and HLA-B27 typing. Because many children with JRA are anemic, a hemoglobin test is often done. If the diagnosis is particularly hard to make, additional tests may be necessary to rule out other diseases.

X-ray examinations of the joints are sometimes helpful early in the course of JRA to find out if some other condition such as a bone infection, tumor, or fracture is causing joint pain and swelling. Later, X-rays may be used to assess joint damage. X-rays of the spine help the doctor to know whether ankylosing spondylitis is present.

A sample of fluid from one or more joints may be aspirated by a needle and examined to find out if there is an infection in the joint. Sometimes the doctor takes a biopsy from a joint or a nodule for examination in the laboratory.

Other diseases, such as psoriasis (chronic skin condition) and colitis (inflammation of the large intestine), can also cause arthritis. These must be ruled out before the doctor reaches a diagnosis of juvenile rheumatoid arthritis.

The parents of a child with joint pain or swelling may be frustrated by the long period of office visits and testing that is sometimes required to pinpoint what is wrong. These procedures, however, are necessary so the physician can be as specific as possible about the child's problems, and so that the treatment can be tailored to fit the condition.

CHOOSING THE DOCTOR AND HEALTH TEAM

Many parents worry about whether they are taking their children to the right doctor. Several different kinds of doctors, including the family physican, internists, or pediatrician, are appropriate—if they are well informed about arthritis in children. The doctor who already knows the child's medical history, including previous illnesses or injuries, is usually the best person to see first.

If the disease is severe or puzzling, the doctor that usually treats the child may refer the parents to a rheumatologist to help with the diagnosis and treatment. Doctors who specialize in JRA are called pediatric rheumatologists.

Sometimes people have difficulty finding a doctor who specializes in JRA. The local county medical society or an accredited hospital in the community can usually help people to locate an appropriate specialist. Local chapters of the Arthritis Foundation can also help in this search.

Other members of the health care team provide special skills that can help a child with JRA. Arthritis clinics and specialized centers exist, where rheumatologists work together with a team of other health professionals to provide total care. The child's regular doctor can help the parents choose such a facility if specialized care is needed.

TREATMENT

Getting a correct diagnosis is really the first step in treating JRA. The treatment program will be based on the kind of arthritis a child has, and the specific symptoms it is causing, and will usually include medications, rest, exercise, eye care, and a balanced diet. Other types of treatment, such as surgery, may be necessary for special long-term problems.

There is no simple, rapid solution to JRA. The treatment is likely to go on for a long time, and progress may seem slow. The treatment chosen by the physician must be followed regularly to help prevent serious joint damage and other problems.

Because the symptoms of a child with JRA can change with time, the parents should expect to have to make some changes periodically in the treatment program.

Medications

Aspirin is the first medication the doctor is likely to prescribe to reduce any pain, inflammation, or fever caused by JRA. About seventy-five percent of children with arthritis need no drug other than aspirin, and children can take considerable amounts of this drug without serious side effects. Because a sufficient blood level of aspirin must be maintained to work against swelling, pain, and stiffness in the joints, most children with arthritis must take large doses of aspirin at least four times each day.

Because of these high doses, the doctor will watch the child carefully for the side effects of too much aspirin. Sometimes the doctor may test the child's blood to make sure the aspirin level is correct. The affected child and its parents should be on the lookout for the warning signs of too much aspirin, so that they can report these signs to the doctor. If the child is in school, its teacher must also know the possible effects of too much aspirin. The warning signs of too much aspirin include:

- Rapid or deep breathing
- Ringing in the ears
- A decrease in hearing
- Drowsiness
- Nausea
- Vomiting
- Irritability
- Unusual behavior

Although several of the nonsteroidal anti-inflammatory drugs are used regularly in treating arthritis in adults, only a few have been approved by the Food and Drug Administration for children. Some are being tested for use in children and may be approved soon. Although the nonsteroidal anti-inflammatory drugs produce fewer side effects than aspirin, they are generally no more effective, and also cost much more than aspirin.

Some children with severe arthritis who aren't helped by aspirin respond to gold treatment. This therapy is usually used only in children with severe polyarticular JRA. Gold treatment is given by injection, usually once a week at first (see page 56). The doctor will watch closely for side effects of the treatment, which can be serious. Four to six months may pass before a child responds to the treatment. Although gold is not effective in all children, when it is, the injections can be continued for many years. Gradually, the injections are given less often.

If aspirin or another nonsteroidal anti-inflammatory drug isn't effective in controlling a child's arthritis, the doctor may try an antimalarial drug. If such a drug is prescribed, the parents should supervise the child closely when he or she takes the medication, and be careful to keep it out of reach of small children. An overdose of this medication can be fatal. Also, because antimalarial drugs can damage the eyes, a child taking one of these drugs should be checked regularly by an ophthalmologist.

Corticosteroid drugs are not often used to treat JRA unless the disease is severe and has not responded to aspirin or other drugs. If corticosteroids are used for long periods—as may be necessary in JRA, particularly the systemic type—their side effects can build up and cause severe problems such as a reduced resistance to infection and high blood pressure.

Doctors try to avoid using corticosteroid drugs in treating JRA because these medications can slow down a child's normal growth, and cause softening of the bones. Since JRA itself can sometimes slow growth and result in a child being smaller than normal, the doctor will try to avoid adding to this potential problem.

If corticosteroid drugs are necessary, the lowest possible dose will generally be used for the shortest length of time.

Penicillamine is an antiarthritic drug that has recently been tested in adults with rheumatoid arthritis and in some children with arthritis. It may be a useful drug for JRA, but is still considered experimental for children.

Exercise

Children with JRA should be encouraged to be reasonably active within the limitations of their disease. They should be allowed to participate in whatever enjoyable play and games their physical condition will allow. Parents in doubt about how much physical activity is right for their child should consult their physician. If exercise seems to aggravate the arthritis or if the child is experiencing a flare-up of the disease, the amount of activity allowed should be restricted.

Play activity may be the only sort of exercise some children need. Others require a certain amount of specially planned exercises to maintain or restore alignment and function of specific joints. The doctor, the nurse, or the physical therapist will teach the parents how the child's joints are supposed to move through their range of motion.

The parents of a school-aged child with JRA may have to discuss with the teacher the child's need to be allowed to walk around the classroom from time to time. Otherwise, the child may become stiff from staying in one position.

A child who has already lost motion in a joint, whose joint has become fixed in a bent position, or whose muscles have become weak may need other exercises. A special therapy program should be worked out by the doctor or physical therapist with the parents and the child.

Although exercise is important for keeping diseased joints from becoming stiff, and for maintaining muscle strength, too much exercise can be harmful. Excessive motion or activity can cause the inflammation in a joint to become worse. Children with JRA can usually tell if they have done too much by the way they feel the next day. The parents must learn to observe the child's reactions carefully, however, because children may not always say how they feel. Sometimes, children with JRA push themselves too hard in trying to keep up with their playmates. On the other hand, they also sometimes learn to use fatigue and soreness to avoid doing activities they don't want to do.

Other Treatment Measures

Depending on the child's condition, other measures than drugs and exercise may be needed to treat JRA. For example, some children benefit from heat or cold treatments. Others need splints to keep certain joints in proper position. These splints have to be adjusted as the child grows and the degree of inflammation changes.

Eye Care

Because JRA sometimes leads to iridocyclitis, eye care must be included in the treatment program. Since the symptoms of this eye disease don't appear until it has already become serious, the best treatment is prevention. Each child should be seen regularly by an ophthalmologist—who is a medical doctor

(M.D.)—rather than by an optometrist, a person who fits glasses. The doctor will explain how often the child should be examined. If iridocyclitis is found early and treated properly, it is unlikely to cause any trouble. If it is allowed to go on, it can result in impaired vision or even blindness.

Eye drops will be prescribed for the child who has irido- cyclitis. One type of eye drops is used to dilate the pupil (enlarge the center black spot). Another type contains a corti- costeroid drug. When corticosteroids are taken in this form, their side effects are not as serious as when these drugs are taken by mouth. If the drops cannot control the iridocyclitis, the child will need to take a corticosteroid in pill form.

Surgery

Surgery is rarely used to treat JRA in its early stages. The only kind of operation that might be considered during that time is a synovectomy, in which inflamed tissue is removed from the synovial lining of the joint. But since the benefit of this operation may last only a year or two, it is not often done.

Orthopedic surgery can play an important role in treating children who have suffered severe joint damage from JRA. Totally replacing an affected joint with an artificial one can reduce pain and improve a child's function. The two joints replaced most successfully are the hip and the knee. Total joint replacement surgery is not generally done until a child has stopped growing. The child usually must be sixteen years old or older before having such an operation. Because these joints ordinarily last only for a given period of time (ten years or less in children), this kind of surgery must be thoroughly discussed in advance among the child, the parents, the family doctor, and the orthopedist before making any decision.

Another operation, called soft-tissue release, may sometimes be used to improve the position of a joint pulled out of line by a contracture. In this operation, the surgeon cuts the tight tissues that caused the contracture, allowing the joint to return to a normal position.

EMOTIONAL CONCERNS

The child with arthritis may develop emotional or behavioral disturbances that its parents cannot deal with alone, and other family members may feel overwhelmed by the difficulties of living with a chronic disease in the family (see Chapter 8). Whatever the case may be, counseling can usually help to work things out. Sometimes all that is needed is a talk with a sympathetic person or someone who is professionally trained to help in these situations.

The doctor, the nurse, or the medical social worker are good sources of help, and can also refer the parents to other sources. Additionally, most local chapters of the Arthritis Foundation provide information about counseling services, parent groups, and other organizations that can help.

THE FUTURE

Juvenile rheumatoid arthritis is a chronic disease. Although most children eventually get well and experience no serious permanent disability from this condition, "eventually" can mean months or years.

In the meantime, the parents and the child must learn to live with the disease. So must everyone else in the family. Families may find it hard to accept that there is no cure for the child's problem. However, the outlook is frequently optimistic for children with JRA; even though no cure is presently available, the disease can usually be controlled.

A remission in JRA may last for months, years, or even forever. However, parents cannot be certain that their child will have a remission. The most important measure is for the family to work with the doctor to manage the disease and keep it under control.

CHAPTER EIGHTEEN

Gout

Many people are surprised to learn that gout belongs to the family of rheumatic diseases. Gout, however, is indeed a form of arthritis. Unlike most other forms, however, it can be controlled completely with proper treatment. Althought the disease cannot be cured, attacks of gout can be prevented. Anyone who follows his or her treatment program closely can avoid the severe pain and unnecessary disability caused by repeated attacks of gout.

AFFECTED POPULATION

An estimated eighty to ninety percent of people with gout are men. The disease is very rare in children and women. The most common age for a first attack is between forty and fifty years old, but gout can start at any age. Women seldom develop gout until after the menopause.

At one time, people considered gout a disease of the wealthy because it seemed to be related to eating rich foods and drinking too much alcohol. Diet and excessive drinking can aggravate gout in those who have gout, but the disease affects people from all walks of life. More than one million people in the United States have it.

PHYSICAL EFFECTS

In gout, certain chemical processes in the body are out of control. One of these affects uric acid, a normal waste product that comes from the breakdown of substances called purines, which are found in many foods as well as in all the cells of the body. Uric acid usually circulates in the blood until it is passed into urine through the kidneys. People with gout have too much uric acid in their blood, a condition called hyperuricemia (although a person can have hyperuricemia without ever getting gout). In people with gout, the uric acid changes into crystals (urate crystals) that deposit in joints and other tissues.

In most people with hyperuricemia, the kidneys do not remove uric acid fast enough from the body. In others, the body

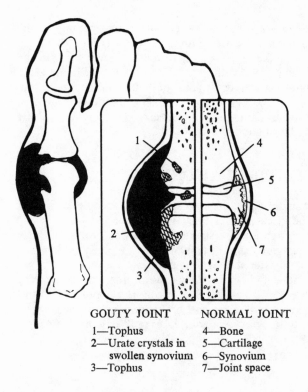

GOUTY JOINT

1—Tophus
2—Urate crystals in
   swollen synovium
3—Tophus

NORMAL JOINT

4—Bone
5—Cartilage
6—Synovium
7—Joint space

Gouty joint vs. normal joint

196

produces too much uric acid. Sometimes both abnormalities are present in the same person. No matter which of these defects is present, numerous urate crystals may eventually (usually after many years) collect in the lining of a joint. Some of these crystals may then fall from the joint lining into the fluid-filled space within the joint or else form in the joint fluid itself. These free urate crystals trigger a severe inflammatory reaction, the acute attack of gouty arthritis. An attack of gout can be triggered by drinking or eating too much, by surgery, by "crash" diets, and occasionally by trauma to a joint.

Although urate crystals can deposit in almost any joint, the big toe is usually the first to be affected, and most people with gout will eventually experience it in the big-toe joint. Joints of the finger, foot, ankle, elbow, wrist, and knee are also subject to attacks of gout. The shoulders, hips, and spine are rarely involved, and only after the person has had attacks in other joints first.

An acute, or sudden attack of gout is extremely painful. The affected joint is obviously inflamed. The skin over the joint turns red or purple and looks shiny, and the joint is swollen and warm. The joint area may be so tender that the slightest touch, even that of a bed sheet, can cause severe pain. The attack usually reaches a peak in a few hours.

These acute attacks usually come on very quickly. Often, a person goes to bed feeling fine and wakes up in the middle of the night with an attack. This kind of sudden attack is different from the way in which the symptoms begin in most other forms of arthritis, which is usually gradual, over a long period.

At first, attacks of gout are usually few and far between and last only a few days. After an attack, everything seems to go back to normal. If the disease is not controlled by medication or diet, the attacks may come more often and last longer. Repeated attacks can damage the affected joint or joints. Between attacks, the person usually feels no symptoms. If one or more joints have been damaged, stiffness and limited joint motion may eventually remain after an attack has subsided.

Urate crystal deposits called tophi or lumps can also occur just under the skin, usually on the outer edge of the ear, over the elbow, or near affected joints. If untreated, these deposits can damage the affected part of the body. They may break through the skin and become infected. They usually don't appear until gout has been present for a long time.

Besides this, uric acid crystals can collect in the urine, forming gravel or stones. This development happens most often in people who pass too little fluid from their bodies. People with gout may have high blood pressure or kidney infections, both of which can cause kidney damage. Thus, the physician must watch for the telltale signs of such damage and begin proper treatment if necessary.

POSSIBLE CAUSES

Physicians now know the direct cause of a gout attack—the presence of urate crystals that cause inflammation—however, there are many factors which can lead to the predisposing of hyperuricemia.

A tendency to hyperuricemia can be inherited. In some people, hyperuricemia is related to alcohol intake and to obesity. It sometimes is a complication of other conditions such as psoriasis or leukemia. Hyperuricemia is sometimes caused by using a number of medications, including diuretics ("water pills"), which are prescribed to get rid of excess body fluid and to lower high blood pressure.

DIAGNOSIS

The doctor examining a patient for gout will take a medical history and then perform a physical examination. A sudden, very painful attack in only one joint often suggests the disease. Some other types of arthritis, however, are similar to gout in some ways, but are not caused by urate crystals. Pseudogout and septic arthritis are two such conditions. The doctor must be sure that the person does not have one of these other forms of arthritis.

One of the tests that will usually be done in an examination for gout is a determination of the amount of uric acid in the blood. As noted earlier, a high level of uric acid doesn't necessarily mean that a person has gout, nor does a normal level mean that gout is definitely not present. The only way to diagnose gout with certainty is for the doctor to remove and examine fluid from an affected joint, and to find urate crystals there.

TREATMENT

Treatment for gout consists primarily of medication and, to some extent, control of the diet. Other than this, anyone with gout should be able to continue his or her normal activities and lifestyle.

Medications

Three kinds of medication are used in treating gout. One category (colchicine, and certain nonsteroidal anti-inflamatory drugs) controls the inflammation of a gouty attack. A second category, uricosuric agents, increases the body's ability to eliminate uric acid by way of the urine, thus lowering the amount of uric acid in the blood. The third kind of medication (allopurinol) decreases uric acid levels in the blood by reducing the rate at which the body produces uric acid.

Of the first category, the drugs used to control inflammation and treat gout attacks, colchicine is the oldest. It has been in use for over 1500 years. An injection of colchicine into a vein at the first sign of pain can bring prompt relief. The drug will also often work if taken by mouth at any time during the first two days of an attack. If the attack has gone on for more than forty-eight hours, colchicine becomes less effective.

Colchicine has several side effects that signal the doctor to lower or discontinue its dose. Diarrhea, nausea, and abdominal cramps can occur when this drug is taken by mouth. If these side effects occur, the person should stop taking the drug and notify the doctor at once.

In addition to its use in controlling acute attacks, colchicine is useful in prevention. A small dose of colchicine taken daily by mouth can help prevent repeated attacks of gout, without causing cramps or diarrhea in people in whom such attacks occur frequently.

Certain nonsteroidal anti-inflammatory drugs, most commonly indomethacin and phenylbutazone, are in the first category of anti-gout drugs. Like colchicine, they rapidly reduce the pain and swelling caused by inflammation. Occasionally, corticosteroids are given by injection directly into an inflamed joint. These drugs are rarely given by mouth in treating gout.

The second category of drugs used for treating gout—the uricosuric agents—helps prevent attacks of the disease by increasing the amount of uric acid passed into the urine. This lowers the level of uric acid in the blood and eventually dissolves the tophi and urate crystals that have been deposited in the tissues lining the joints. These medicines have no effect in treating an attack of gout, and may even make the acute attack worse.

The two uricosuric drugs commonly used for gout are probenecid (Benemid) and sulfinpyrazone (Anturane). In order to be effective, these drugs must be taken every day. The doctor will check the level of uric acid in the blood from time to time, and the dosage of whichever uricosuric agent is being used may be changed if necessary. When a normal level of uric acid is reached, no more urate crystals will be deposited, and those already present will start dissolving.

One side effect of both probenecid and sulfinpyrazone is that when first given, they can increase the risk of kidney stones by increasing the uric acid content of the urine. An important point is that aspirin should not be taken with either probenecid or sulfinpyrazone, since it blocks the action of these drugs on the kidney.

The third category of anti-gout drug consists of the single drug allopurinol. Like the uricosuric drugs, allopurinol is used to prevent attacks of gout, but rather than increasing the body's excretion of uric acid, it changes the way in which the body produces uric acid, decreasing the amount of uric acid in both the blood and the urine. Allopurinol can also be very effective in dissolving tophi. It is the best drug for people whose kidneys are not normal or whose urine contains too much uric acid, causing kidney stones. The drug does, however, have a number of undesirable side effects, particularly skin rashes, lowering of the blood count, and severe allergy.

With these different kinds of drugs, gout can be controlled in a variety of ways. Also, some people have attacks of gout more often when they start taking drugs which lower blood uric acid levels. This may occur because as urate crystals already in the joints start to dissolve, the remaining crystals in the joint lining may break off and cause inflammation more easily. These attacks can be prevented by taking small daily doses of colchicine. Eventually, when the crystals in the joint lining have all dissolved, the attacks will stop.

People who have high blood levels of uric acid, or who have tophi, may need to take one of the uricosuric drugs or allopurinol to reduce their uric acid levels. The doctor may also want such a person to take colchicine or another drug that reduces inflammation, since such treatment can bring on attacks of gout. This reaction tends to happen when the uric acid content of the blood is lowered very rapidly.

To be effective in lowering uric acid levels, the uricosuric drugs or allopurinol must be taken continuously. Not all people with gout require these drugs; whether a person takes them depends on the judgment of the doctor and the person's willingness to make a lifelong commitment to take daily medications.

Many people with gout are taught by their doctors how to begin treatment on their own, should an acute attack of gout begin. The doctor may suggest that the person keep a supply of colchicine or another anti-inflammatory drug on hand to take at the first sign of an attack.

As when starting any new drug, the person who will be taking drugs for gout should tell the physician of all other drugs he or she is taking, including diuretics and nonprescription drugs such as aspirin. Some of the gout medications will not work properly if other drugs are being taken at the same time.

Diet

Myths abound concerning the relationship between diet and gout. Here are the facts:

1. A person who is overweight should develop a weight-loss program under the doctor's supervision. The person should not fast or try to diet too severely, or the gout may become worse temporarily because the level of uric acid in the blood may rise.
2. Because a few foods tend to raise the uric acid level in the blood, the physician may caution a person with gout to avoid eating them. These foods include organ meats such as kidneys, liver, and sweetbreads, as well as sardines, anchovies, and meat extracts (Table 3). Usually, people who have gout can eat what they like in moderation, but should discuss the details of their diet with the physician.
3. A person with gout does not need to avoid coffee and tea. Alcohol consumed in moderation (i.e., about two ounces of hard liquor, a can of beer, or a glass of wine per day) is permitted. Too much alcohol may be

Table 3: RELATIVE PURINE CONTENT OF COMMON FOODS

Group A: (Foods containing a high purine concentration, about 150 to 1,000 milligrams per 100 grams.)

Liver	Gravies
Sweetbreads	Broths
Brains	Mussels
Fish roe	Wine
Beer	Anchovies
Kidney	Heart
Sardines	Herring

Group B: (Foods containing moderate amounts of purine, 50 to 150 milligrams per 100 grams, which the physician usually limits to one serving each day.)

Meats	Mushrooms
Peas	Spinach
Cauliflower	Whole grain cereals
Lentils	Fowl
Yeast	Fish (except as noted above)
Beans	
Asparagus	Other seafoods

Group C: (Foods containing negligible amounts of purine, which are not subject to limitation.)

Vegetables (except as noted above)
Fruits
Milk
Cheese
Eggs
Spices and condiments, including salt and vinegar
Refined cereals and cereal products
Butter and fats (in moderation)
Sugar and sweets
Vegetable soups (clear)
Nuts

associated with hyperuricemia, and can bring on a gout attack.

4. A high daily intake of nonalcoholic fluids is recommended (a minimum of two quarts), especially in people who have had kidney stones.

Surgery

Surgery is rarely used to treat gout. People who have large tophi that are draining, infected, or interfering with joint movements may need to have these tophi removed surgically. If gout has caused severe disability or crippling, several kinds of operation can be done to relieve pain and improve the function of the affected joints (see Chapter 7). After surgery on gouty tophi or joints, the healing is sometimes very slow.

THE FUTURE

The person with gout may have no more than a few mild attacks in his or her entire lifetime. More commonly, however, the attacks occur increasingly often if the disease is not treated. This repeated series of attacks may lead to disability and chronic pain.

People with very high uric acid levels in their blood may develop kidney stones. Other problems with the kidneys may develop slowly, and tests of kidney function may be needed from time to time.

Many of these effects can be avoided by seeing a doctor early in the course of gout and following the treatment program. The first few attacks of gout do no permanent damage; a complete recovery can be expected, with perfectly normal joints. When a person has repeated attacks in a joint, however, enough urate crystals are deposited to cause damage. This damage is entirely avoidable if the person keeps the gout under control. Those who do control their gout can look forward to normal lives with no permanent effects from the disease.

CHAPTER NINETEEN

Pseudogout (Calcium Pyrophosphate Dihydrate Crystal Deposition Disease)

Calcium pyrophosphate dihydrate crystal deposition disease (CPPD disease) is a tongue-twisting name for a disease that has been recognized as a cause of arthritis only since 1962. It results from deposits of a certain kind of calcium crystal in joints. Because the disease is chronic, it often produces repeated attacks of pain and swelling for many years. However, CPPD disease can usually be controlled with proper treatment.

This disease may take different forms. Since the CPPD crystals may deposit in cartilage, where they can be seen on an X-ray, the condition is sometimes called "chondrocalcinosis," the Latin term for "calcium in the cartilage." In some people, the CPPD crystals may cause acute attacks of severe pain in a single joint, which can resemble gout. Such individuals are said to have "pseudogout" because gout also results from crystals—in this case uric acid crystals rather than CPPD crystals—deposited in the joints.

In both pseudogout and gout, crystals leak into the joint to cause inflammation and sudden dramatic pain and swelling. The most common joint to be affected in gout is the joint in the big toe; in pseudogout, the knee is most often affected. Acute attacks of either gout or CPPD disease commonly occur after surgery or some injury.

Much of the confusion over identifying CPPD disease as a specific disease came about because some people with it also have other forms of joint disease such as osteoarthritis (see Chapter 10) and rheumatoid arthritis (see Chapter 11). But

CPPD disease is distinct from these others, and people with CPPD disease and another rheumatic disease need treatment for both conditions.

One condition that often occurs together with CPPD disease is osteoarthritis, probably because most people with CPPD disease are elderly, and osteoarthritis is also common in older people. It is often difficult to determine how much joint pain is due to CPPD disease and how much to osteoarthritis.

AFFECTED POPULATION

CPPD disease occurs mainly in older people. The average age of onset is in the middle sixties, and it rarely occurs in people under thirty. The disease affects an equal number of men and women.

PHYSICAL EFFECTS

CPPD disease appears in different forms in different people. About one-fourth of all people affected with the disease have sudden attacks in which swelling and pain develop rapidly in a joint (pseudogout). The joint becomes hot and stiffened. The skin over the affected joint often turns red. The attack usually reaches its peak within twelve to thirty-six hours and lasts for several days, sometimes weeks. In most people, the symptoms of an acute attack will eventually go away even without treatment.

The milder, more chronic, forms of CPPD disease are more likely to occur in several joints at the same time, such as the wrists and fingers, as well as the knee. The pain and swelling aren't as severe as in a sudden attack, but last longer. The pain usually becomes worse during or after activity. Some people with this chronic form have acute attacks also. Others with the chronic form never have an acute attack.

Most people with either acute or chronic CPPD disease do have periods when they have no symptoms at all.

POSSIBLE CAUSES

The direct cause of the symptoms of CPPD disease is the deposition of CPPD crystals in the joint. This causes a painful inflammatory reaction that is the body's attempt to get rid of the CPPD crystals. As part of this reaction, many white cells invade the affected joint from the blood, causing it to swell and hurt.

Scientists are not sure what originally causes the body to form the CPPD crystals that cause the disease. Though the crystals contain calcium, consuming milk or other foods high in calcium has nothing to do with the disease. Medical researchers are finding many clues, however, to different causes of CPPD disease. Pyrophosphate is produced by many different tissues but is ordinarily broken down rapidly by the body. Scientists think that people who have CPPD disease are either making too much pyrophosphate in the cartilage or do not eliminate it quickly enough to prevent it from building up. There are several kinds of CPPD disease, and one rare form is known to be inherited. In some people, CPPD disease is linked to another underlying disease. For example, an overactive parathyroid gland can cause CPPD disease. The parathyroid gland produces a hormone that regulates the body's calcium level in the same manner a thermostat in a house controls the heat level. In the conditions termed hyperparathyroidism ("hyper" means more than normal), overactivity of the parathyroid gland causes too much calcium to build up in the body; this calcium may form crystals by combining with pyrophosphate.

Hypothyroidism ("hypo" means less than normal) may also be related to CPPD disease. In this condition, the thyroid gland produces too little of its hormone, causing most people to feel sluggish and apathetic. The crystals probably form in cartilage as a result of low levels of thyroid hormone, but attacks of pain and swelling of the joints do not occur until the condition is diagnosed and treated with thyroid hormone replacement.

CPPD disease has been found to occur in some people with diabetes mellitus (a disease in which there is a defect in regulating sugar in the body), high blood pressure, and atherosclerosis (hardening of the arteries). Other people with CPPD disease have too much iron (hemochromatosis), too much copper (Wilson's disease), or not enough magnesium in their blood.

Some people have had severe attacks of CPPD disease soon after being injured, after surgery, or after any acute body stress such as heart attack.

DIAGNOSIS

The doctor's first step in making a diagnosis of CPPD disease will be to ask questions about the symptoms and to perform a physical examination. The doctor will pay close attention to the joints, and look for signs that could indicate another disease associated with CPPD disease.

If you are having an attack, the doctor will remove some of the joint fluid to see if it contains CPPD crystals. X-rays of the affected joints will usually show whether CPPD crystals are present, and whether the cartilage has been damaged as a result. The doctor will usually order certain blood tests to help rule out other kinds of arthritis and identify any of the diseases. For example, the doctor may want to determine the calcium and phosphorus levels in the blood to see whether hyperparathyroidism exists, to check the iron levels in the blood to learn whether hemochromatosis is present, and to test for the level of thyroid hormone to seek evidence of hypothyroidism.

TREATMENT

The treatment program for CPPD disease is designed individually because it depends on how severe the disease is and whether the person also has another illness or another kind of arthritis in addition. Most likely, the program will involve some combination of joint aspiration, medication, rest, special exercises, and protection of the joints. Rarely, surgery may be advised. During an acute attack, the goal of treatment is to relieve the painful symptoms. The goals of long-term treatment are to keep the illness under control and retain good function of the affected joints.

Joint Aspiration

For acute attacks, the doctor will probably remove, or aspirate, some fluid from the affected joint. Such joint aspiration is not only valuable for diagnosing CPPD disease, but also to remove many of the CPPD crystals causing the pain and inflammation. Sometimes the doctor will inject a corticosteroid directly into the joint.

Medication

The drugs used most often in treating CPPD disease are the nonsteroidal anti-inflammatory drugs (NSAIDs). They reduce the pain and swelling caused by inflammation. They are very effective for treating acute attacks of CPPD disease, and usually produce relief within a few days. For people who have peptic ulcers, treatment with intravenous colchicine as used in gout may be very helpful. Giving this anti-inflammatory drug intravenously circumvents the irritation to the stomach that may be caused by NSAID use.

Less often, doctors prescribe aspirin for CPPD attacks. Whether prescribing an NSAID or aspirin, the doctor may lower the dosage once the attack subsides, but continue the medication to control the illness, especially if it is chronic. Some people eventually won't need to continue any medication at all; others will need to keep taking medication to reduce the risk of future problems.

Rest and Exercise

During an attack, the affected joint needs to be rested. Occasionally splints are recommended for resting and protecting joints subject to repeated attacks. Splints, canes, and other devices used for protecting joints should be fitted by experts, such as physical or occupational therapists.

Once the acute attack subsides, or if the disease exists only in its mild, chronic form, rest should be balanced with exercise. The doctor or physical therapist can help plan the proper kind of exercise to build muscle strength and retain full motion of the affected joints.

Surgery

In a very few people with CPPD disease, surgery may be necessary for a joint that is badly damaged, very painful, or unstable. Surgeons usually replace such a joint with an artificial one made of plastic and metal (see Chapter 7). The joints most often requiring surgery are the knees, hips, and shoulders.

THE FUTURE

Most people with CPPD disease find that it does not prevent them from continuing their normal lives. Because there is no permanent cure, many people will need to continue their treatment programs, even during periods of remission, in order to maintain control over the pain and inflammation the disease causes. Unless there has been serious damage to the joints, most people can participate in their usual activities, with minor restrictions during flare-ups.

In the relatively short time since CPPD disease was identified, researchers have made progress in distinguishing CPPD disease from many other diseases it resembles and in determining what other diseases increase one's rate of developing CPPD disease. Concern is now focused on finding out how and where the CPPD crystals are formed and whether they result from chemical defects in the body. Most likely, several different causes of CPPD will be found.

CHAPTER TWENTY

Infectious Arthritis

Infectious arthritis is a form of arthritis brought on by infection due to bacteria, viruses, or fungi.

Unlike most rheumatic diseases, many forms of infectious arthritis are curable and leave no long-term effects. Infectious arthritis usually comes on suddenly, and requires immediate treatment. Without prompt treatment, infection can seriously damage the involved joints and might spread to other parts of the body.

AFFECTED POPULATION

Just as anyone can catch a cold or the flu, anyone can get infectious arthritis. But some people cannot handle infection normally, putting them more at risk. People for whom there is a high risk of infection include people with chronic alcoholism and those who abuse drugs. Medical problems such as diabetes, sickle-cell anemia, kidney disease, immune deficiency, and some forms of cancer can also increase the risk of infection. Additionally, infants and elderly people have more trouble fighting off infections. Certain drugs such as corticosteroids and the cytotoxic agents often used to treat cancer also decrease the body's resistance to infection. People who already have some kind of arthritis, particularly rheumatoid arthritis, are prone to get infections in the involved joints.

TYPES OF INFECTIOUS ARTHRITIS

Bacteria

Gonococcus

Gonorrhea is the most common bacterial cause of arthritis, but differs from the others in several ways. People who develop this condition are usually young people who do not fit into any of the categories of decreased resistance of infection described above. It is more common in women than in men, probably because women have fewer symptoms when they develop gonorrhea so that treatment is delayed and the gonococci (the bacteria) have more time to enter the bloodstream and subsequently the joints. Infectious arthritis usually develops a few days to a week or more after the person first notices the discharge from the vagina or penis characteristic of gonorrhea. In many people, however, no discharge is noticed. Often the person develops a fever, sometimes with chils, and a rash consisting of a few red, dime-sized spots that are raised in the center. Inflammation of the tendons is common. The arthritis may develop in one or two joints, most often the knees or wrists. If not treated promptly, the infection can cause serious damage to joints.

Staphylococci, Streptococci, and Pneumococci

These Gram-positive bacteria (so-called because of the way they appear through a microscope after exposure to the Gram strain) are—after gonococci—the main causes of acute infectious arthritis. Usually some other infection is also present such as meningitis, pneumonia, or an abscess, often no other site of infection is evident.

E. Coli, Pseudomonas, and Proteus

These are the most common Gram-negative infections. They are less apt to produce arthritis than the Gram-positive organisms. They often arise from kidney or bowel infection and attack people with an immune system that has been weakened by another illness.

Tuberculosis

This organism and a group of similar bacteria called atypical mycobacteria were a very important cause of arthritis forty years ago but are much less of a threat today. They usually involve only one joint, but the arthritis is very slow to develop and often the correct diagnosis is made only after the joint has suffered serious injury.

Tuberculosis or any of the fungal infections can be accompanied by an acute painful arthritis called erythema nodosum, which often attacks the ankles and other joints. The name refers to the reddish, tender nodules—about the size of a quarter —that develop under the skin of the lower legs. The bacteria or fungi are not actually present in either the skin or the joints. Erythema nodosum seems to be an unusual reaction of the body to certain infections or other causes of inflammation.

Lyme Disease

Lyme Disease is a form of infectious arthritis resulting from a tick bite. The bite can sometimes be recognized by the red rash that surrounds it. The tick carries a type of bacterium called a spirochete, which it injects into the bloodstream when it bites. The spirochete may travel to joints, the brain, and the heart, where it causes an acute inflammation accompanied by fever, chills, and soreness all over the body. Though the attack usually subsides by itself, it can flare up again several times over a year or more if it is not properly treated with an antibiotic.

Others

Almost any bacterium that can infect people can cause arthritis. In young children, Hemophilus influenza, which rarely affects adults, is a major cause of infectious arthritis.

Fungi

Fungi do not often produce arthritis and when they do, the infection usually spreads to the joint from one of the bones forming the joint rather than via the bloodstream. This form of arthritis develops very slowly, and is similar to that caused by tuberculosis. Bird droppings, especially from chickens and pigeons, are frequent carriers of two types of fungal infections: histoplasmosis and cryptococcosis. Sporotrichosis is apt to attack gardeners and florists because the fungi grow on certain plants, especially roses. Blastomycosis occurs mainly in the southeastern states and coccidiodomycosis in the San Joaquin Valley of California.

Viruses

Viruses usually produce an acute arthritis that nearly always goes away without treatment. Arthritis is a frequent early symptom in one type of infectious hepatitis. By the time the individual develops the jaundice characteristic of the illness, the arthritis has disappeared. German measles (rubella) commonly produces a form of arthritis that can occasionally last as long as a year after the rash is gone. Vaccination with German measles vaccine can sometimes cause arthritis. Mumps and infectious mononucleosis are two other viral diseases that can lead to acute arthritis.

PHYSICAL EFFECTS

Infectious arthritis usually spreads to a joint through the bloodstream. Sometimes, however, an infectious agent enters the joint directly through a wound or from a nearby abscess. Rarely, an infection may develop in a joint after fluid has been drained from it. Occasionally, an infecting agent shows up in the joint for no apparent reason. Presumably it entered the body through the skin, the throat, or some other route and traveled directly to the joint via the bloodstream. Once they multiply there, white cells enter the joint from the blood to fight the infection, resulting in a painful, inflamed joint.

The symptoms of infectious arthritis depend on the nature of the agent and the general health of the person affected. Most often, bacteria are responsible and the symptoms develop quickly. These symptoms include fever, weakness, headaches, and aching throughout the body. Soon the affected joint or joints usually become very painful, swollen, red, and stiff. Most people also have chills, and become very sick indeed.

Infectious arthritis usually affects only one joint, although it occasionally involves more than one. Those most often involved are large ones: the knees, ankles, shoulders, hips, elbows, and wrists. For people who already have some form of arthritis, especially rheumatoid arthritis, the infection resembles a flare-up of the basic disease. For this reason, anyone with arthritis must tell his or her doctor immediately upon noticing sudden pain, swelling, heat, or redness in a joint, since it may mean an infection.

DIAGNOSIS

In diagnosing infectious arthritis, the doctor asks detailed questions about the symptoms and about anything that may explain the person's condition, such as recent injuries or the presence of other infectious diseases. It is vital to be completely truthful with the physician when discussing sexual exposures, including homosexual contacts, which are a common way of transmitting gonorrhea.

The diagnostic process includes a complete physical examination and several tests such as X-rays and blood tests. The doctor will usually remove some fluid from the infected joint and examine it under the microscope and by culturing it to identify the specific infection present. Tests of the joint fluid can also yield other diagnostic clues; for example, if the sugar content of the fluid is low or the number of white blood cells is very high, an infection is probably the cause.

Besides these tests, the physician may remove a small bit of tissue from the joint, performing a joint biopsy. The biopsied tissue will then be examined with a microscope and by culture to look for infectious agents. Chronic infections such as tuberculosis and those caused by most fungi are often diagnosed by this method. Cultures may also be taken from other sources such as blood, urine, the vagina, and skin, which may be the origin of infection.

Other tests may be needed to find out where the infection originated. These tests may take a few days to complete, but the infection may be potentially serious enough that the doctor will begin treatment before all of the test results are known. When infectious arthritis is suspected, hospitalization is usually necessary.

TREATMENT

The specific treatment for infectious arthritis depends on which agent is causing the disease and on the condition of the person who has it. The program is designed first to eradicate the infection and then to get rid of the arthritis that developed along with it. It is often a combination of medication, pain control, drainage of joints, and later, follow-up physical therapy.

Medication and Joint Drainage

Infectious arthritis caused by bacteria, is treated with an antibiotic. The specific antibiotic used depends on the bacterium causing the disease, since different antibiotics are required to destroy different bacteria. When the infecting organism has been isolated from the joint by culture, its susceptibility to different antibiotics can be tested in the laboratory. This step is important because all strains of a single type of bacterium such as the staphylococcus are not equally susceptible to the same antibiotics. The antibiotic used to treat the disease may be given to the person intravenously (directly into the veins) to achieve high blood levels or by injection into the muscles. Some people need to take an antibiotic only for a week or two. Others may need it for several months, especially if the infection is caused by tuberculosis or a fungus.

The doctor may prescribe anti-inflammatory drugs such as aspirin, especially if the arthritis is caused by a virus, since antibiotics have no effect on viral diseases.

The treatment of infectious arthritis may also include repeated drainage of the joint(s) either by a needle or by an operation with insertion of a drain. Joint drainage is performed to remove harmful enzymes and other chemicals that are released by infecting bacteria and by the body's own white cells which can destroy the cartilage. At first, the doctor may drain the joint every day. During the treatment period, the doctor will repeat the tests of blood and joint fluid to find out how fast the organism is being eliminated. At some point, the doctor may be able to begin giving the medication in the form of pills rather than injections, allowing the person to be treated at home. However, some antibiotics such as those used to treat fungi can be given only intravenously. It is vital to keep taking them as long as the doctor advises, in order to prevent the disease from recurring. If they are stopped too early, there is a danger that the infectious agent will develop resistance to the drug. If the infection then returns, some other, less effective drug may have to be used the second time.

Joint Rest and Protection

In the early stages of infectious arthritis, resting and protecting the infected joint(s) may be an important part of the treatment program. Resting splints may be used to limit movement so that the joint tissues will not be damaged. The doctor will recommend when to resume movement of the joints.

Physical Therapy

As the infection is controlled, the doctor may prescribe certain exercises to build up muscle strength and prevent loss of motion. They may include exercises in which the joints are moved gently in all of their normal directions, exercises done with the help of a therapist, and exercises done at home to increase muscle strength. Gradually, the person will be able to resume normal activity.

THE FUTURE

If an infection that spreads to the joints is diagnosed and treated early, there will usually be no lasting joint damage. Once the infection has been stopped with drugs or by the natural defenses of the body, the affected joints should return to normal when the proper therapy program is followed.

Sometimes infectious arthritis results in permanent joint damage. Occasionally surgery may help restore function in these joints.

CHAPTER TWENTY-ONE

Psoriatic Arthritis

For more than 150 years, physicians have recognized a connection between the chronic skin disease known as psoriasis and arthritis. Many people have psoriasis, which causes scaly red patches on the body, especially on the scalp, elbows, knees, and neck. Like everyone else, people with psoriasis may also develop any one of the variety of different rheumatic diseases. But arthritis can be directly related to psoriasis, and is therefore called psoriatic arthritis.

In most people with psoriatic arthritis, the symptoms of arthritis are mild and require little or no treatment. In a very few, the arthritis can be severe. Whether severe or mild, psoriatic arthritis should be diagnosed accurately so that proper treatment can be started when needed.

AFFECTED POPULATION

Of the Americans who have psoriasis, only five to eight percent get psoriatic arthritis. The arthritis is more common in women than men, and usually occurs between the ages of twenty and thirty, although it can occur at any age in either sex.

PHYSICAL EFFECTS

Scientists are unsure whether psoriatic arthritis is a single disease or a group of related disorders. There are three major forms of this arthritis, all of which may cause only minimum discomfort.

In the most common form, only a few joints, usually fingers and toes, are affected. The involved joints are frequently very enlarged and the fingers or toes so swollen that they have been given the name "sausage digits." In a second type, "classical psoriatic arthritis," the joints at the ends of the fingers (next to the nails) are inflamed, and the fingernails become thickened and pitted from psoriasis. This form may attack any other joints except the spine.

The third type of psoriatic arthritis occurs primarily in the spine, causing the condition known as spondylitis (see Chapter 15). The sacroiliac and lumbar joints at the base of the spine are affected, and the symptoms are the same as those of ankylosing spondylitis. Some people with this type of psoriatic arthritis eventually do develop typical ankylosing spondylitis.

Other joints may develop arthritis as well. In particular, people with psoriasis and spinal arthritis can develop an arthritis of the fingers in which both bone and joints are destroyed so that the fingers telescope (so-called "main en lorgnette"). Some people with psoriasis develop arthritis of many joints in symmetrical fashion (i.e., the same joint on both sides of the body). This pattern resembles that of rheumatoid arthritis, making it difficult to distinguish true rheumatoid arthritis in a person with psoriasis from psoriatic arthritis. If the latex test for rheumatoid arthritis is positive or if X-rays reveal the characteristic damage of rheumatoid arthritis, the diagnosis of rheumatoid arthritis can be established by the physician. Sometimes there is no way to be sure which is present.

The major symptoms of psoriatic arthritis are soreness of the fingers or other joints. Sometimes one or two fingers will swell up in the shape of sausages. If the spine is affected, backache is common. Aside from joint pain, people with psoriatic arthritis usually feel well.

Even though there is no permanent cure for either psoriasis or psoriatic arthritis, either or both may go away spontaneously. After a few months or years of active disease, several years may pass with no symptoms. After this the rash, joint pain, or back pain may come back again for a variable length of time. The severity of the skin disease and the joint disease tend to parallel each other. If the rash flares up in a person with psoriasis who has had arthritis in the past, the arthritis will probably soon flare up as well.

POSSIBLE CAUSES

The cause of psoriasis and the arthritis that accompanies it is not yet known. Scientists have found a marked increase in the blood supply of the skin and in the growth and death of skin cells in people with psoriasis.

The development of psoriasis, like ankylosing spondylitis and rheumatoid arthritis (Chapter 2), does seem to be related to certain inherited HLA markers. Several markers have been implicated. People with psoriasis who develop the sacroiliac and spinal arthritis of ankylosing spondylitis frequently have the HLA-B27 marker characteristic of that disease. So far, none of the markers found in psoriasis has been associated with any special type of joint disease. When more than one person in a family develops psoriasis, it probably results from inheriting a genetic tendency to develop the disease.

DIAGNOSIS

Before making a diagnosis, the doctor will go through a number of steps to determine the type of psoriatic arthritis that is present. The relationship between the skin condition and the joint symptoms is important. The physician may ask such questions as, "Do these symptoms get better when the skin clears? Does the joint pain remain when the skin is better, or the other way around?" Also, the doctor will want to know about psoriasis and arthritis, particularly ankylosing spondylitis, in the family.

Blood tests may be done to see if rheumatoid factor is present. The uric acid level of the blood may be high in psoriasis, but it rarely—if ever—produces gout. If the disease has existed for more than a year, X-rays may show bone changes that could help in making a diagnosis.

In the physical examination, the doctor looks for signs of

the most typical form of psoriatic arthritis, especially redness and swelling of the small joints at the ends of the fingers (the distal interphalangeal joints) in conjunction with thickened, pitted yellowish nails. In the most common form of psoriatic arthritis, finding a single finger swollen in the shape of a sausage, a condition called dactylitis, is helpful in making the diagnosis.

People with sacroiliac joint inflammation will usually complain of pain in the lower back. There may be swelling or inflammation in the large joints of the arms and legs, and sometimes shortening of the fingers if they are severely involved.

Once a diagnosis of psoriatic arthritis has been made, further blood tests or X-rays are rarely needed. An exception to this occurs in the case of severe disease or if a person who is receiving certain kinds of treatment which require the procedures may have to be repeated from time to time.

TREATMENT

Depending on the severity of the illness, the treatment of psoriatic arthritis may include measures to keep the skin condition under control, medications for the joints, and special programs of exercise. Since this is a chronic disease, it will require attention over the years.

Medication

Different medications are usually used for the skin problems and joint problems in psoriatic arthritis, although successful treatment of the skin may benefit the joints as well. If the joints are only mildly affected, medication may not be needed. If the arthritis appears to be getting worse or the pain in the joints interferes with daily living, the person may be given a prescription for one of the nonsteroidal anti-inflammatory drugs. These drugs may have to be taken for a few days, for weeks or months, or for a longer time, depending on the course of the illness. Aspirin, which is useful in treating rheumatoid arthritis, is not always as effective as NSAIDs against psoriatic arthritis.

The corticosteroids are seldom used—and only under exceptional circumstances—in psoriatic arthritis. Steroids taken by mouth can have serious side effects, and many doctors feel that their side effects outweigh their benefits in the disease, and, after withdrawal, may cause the psoriasis to become worse. Injections of steroids into individual joints, however, are helpful for some people.

Gold injections and hydroxychloroquine (Plaquenil) are often beneficial in psoriatic as well as rheumatoid arthritis.

Rarely, psoriatic arthritis can be progressive and cause severe joint damage. If this happens, immunosuppressive drugs, usually methotrexate, may be given. These drugs are effective against both the skin condition and the joint problems of psoriatic arthritis and may be given by mouth or by injection. People receiving these drugs need to have frequent blood tests to be sure no serious side effects are developing. Liver damage is the most serious side effect of methotrexate. It can be detected only by blood tests. Occasionally a liver biopsy (performed with a special needle introduced through the skin) may be performed to determine if the liver has been injured by the drug.

Rest and Exercise

The proper amount of rest and exercise in psoriatic arthritis depends upon the person who has the disease and upon its severity. Joints that hurt can become stiff from lack of use. The doctor may recommend certain exercises to maintain the range of motion of the affected joints and to strengthen the muscles that move them. A physical therapist can design an individualized exercise program.

If the joints receive particular stress because of the person's type of employment—as the finger joints do for a person who does much typing, or the shoulders or hips in someone who does heavy lifting—the person may need to modify his or her job or change to another type of work to protect the stressed joints. Joints that are affected by arthritis should be protected from injury and overwork.

Otherwise, most people with psoriatic arthritis should be able to continue to live as they did before the disease developed. Since psoriatic arthritis only rarely causes the fatigue seen in some other forms of arthritis, a normal amount of rest and sleep is adequate.

Surgery

Joints that are severely damaged by psoriatic arthritis can be replaced surgically, although surgery is seldom necessary in this disease, since the hips and knees are usually not involved. As noted elsewhere in this book, surgical operations to replace diseased joints have become very successful in recent years.

THE FUTURE

Most people with psoriatic arthritis can live nearly normal lives with little disruption. Because the condition is chronic, however, it requires some continuing care and monitoring, with the treatment being adjusted during flare-ups or periods of remission. Relatively few people develop serious joint deformity from this disease.

CHAPTER TWENTY-TWO

Polymyalgia Rheumatica and Giant-Cell (Temporal) Arteritis

Polymyalgia rheumatica (PMR) is a rheumatic disorder, which means it involves tendons, muscles, and other tissues around the joints. In PMR, these structures become stiff and painful, often severely so.

The name of the disease describes it: "poly" means many, "myo" means muscle, "algia" means pain, and "rheumatica" refers to an inflammation of connective tissue, such as muscle and ligaments.

Although PMR can last for months or years, it almost always goes away eventually. Most often, PMR lasts about two years, but it can last from a few months to many years.

Some people with PMR also have a condition called giant-cell arteritis, which is described later in this chapter. This is an illness that affects some of the body's arteries. Like polymyalgia, it, too, responds well to prompt treatment.

Because it affects older people, many people mistakenly attribute the symptoms to the effects of old age. Because this illness can usually be treated successfully, prompt medical care is important for relief of the symptoms of pain and stiffness and prevention of serious complications. Almost all people with PMR can resume their usual activities if they follow their prescribed treatment programs and keep a positive attitude about their condition.

AFFECTED POPULATION

Most people with PMR are more than fifty years old, usually considerably older. The disease affects white people more frequently than members of any other race, and occurs more often in women than in men. Most people with PMR have previously been active and healthy.

PHYSICAL EFFECTS

The major symptoms of PMR are pain and stiffness in the neck, shoulders, upper arms, lower back, hips, and thighs. The symptoms often come on quickly, and the stiffness is most severe in the morning. In some people, however, the symptoms come on very gradually, and it is hard to tell exactly when they began. Some people report going to bed feeling fine but waking up the next morning feeling as if they had done heavy physical work. The morning stiffness can be so bad that even getting out of bed may be difficult. Many people with PMR find they need help from a family member to get out of bed in the morning, or have to use a chair or nightstand to help themselves stand up. Difficulty in moving may also occur after long periods of sitting still.

The pain of PMR is symmetrical, occurring on both sides of the body. It is hard for some people to pinpoint the location of the pain when describing it to the doctor, but most say it hurts more in the muscles than in the joints, and that they generally feel run-down and miserable.

Pain at night is common in PMR. Most people with the disease feel comfortable when they lie still in bed, but moving around or turning over may cause them discomfort.

Other symptoms of PMR are usually mild. They include sweating at night, a slight fever, lack of appetite, a little swelling in one or two joints, loss of energy, fatigue, and depression.

POSSIBLE CAUSES

The cause of PMR is not known. Because the disease is most common in white people, and sometimes two or more members of the same family have PMR, some scientists think that it may be at least partly inherited. So far this hypothesis has not been proven. Researchers have not been able to find any evidence that it is contagious.

The blood of many people with active PMR contains material that appears to be antibodies linked to some antigen. This evidence suggests that some kind of unusual immune response may occur in the disease. Antibodies have also been found in the diseased arteries of people with PMR and the related condition known as giant-cell arteritis. Scientists, however, do not yet know what the presence of these antibodies means.

DIAGNOSIS

The diagnosis of PMR may require several visits to the doctor. Because the symptoms of this illness are similar to those of several other diseases that affect the joints and muscles, the doctor will often test for these diseases. He or she will ask detailed questions about the symptoms and perform a physical examination, looking for any clues to explain the pain.

The doctor will also take a blood sample for several tests. The most valuable test is the erythrocyte sedimentation rate, since people with PMR usually have much higher sedimentation values than those of other people of the same age.

To exclude the presence of the muscle disease known as polymyositis, the doctor may perform a muscle biopsy—a procedure in which a small bit of muscle is removed and then examined with a microscope. In PMR, the muscle appears normal, while in polymyositis and certain other muscle diseases the muscles show damage. People with polymyositis also have higher-than-normal levels of certain enzymes in their blood, whereas the levels of these enzymes are normal in PMR.

TREATMENT

Although there is no single specific laboratory test for diagnosing PMR, the response to treatment is usually so good that it helps prove whether the diagnosis was right or wrong.

The most effective drugs for this disease are the corticosteroids. Most people receive prednisone. This treatment usually results in marked improvement within a few days.

As the disease diminishes, the doctor usually lowers the

dosage of prednisone gradually and then keeps it at a maintenance level for some time. This drug maintenance treatment is necessary even when the person with PMR feels fine, because it will help prevent flare-ups. The length of the maintenance period can last up to several years, depending on the person's condition and response to the drug. Because of the potential for drug side effects, which are more serious in the elderly, doctors closely follow people being treated with corticosteroid drugs, even though the dosage is low.

Not everyone who has PMR will need to take corticosteroids. Some may do well on aspirin or a nonsteroidal drug. Taking aspirin regularly for a while after the symptoms have disappeared may prevent flare-ups until the disease has completely stopped.

During any period of pain and stiffness, people with PMR have to avoid being either too active or not active enough. Either extreme will increase the pain and stiffness caused by the disease. During painful episodes, people with the disease should rest more during the day than when they are feeling well, but should also try to avoid long periods without movement. Once the drug therapy starts working, activity can be increased. The treatment program does not require special exercises; the person's usual activity should be enough.

GIANT-CELL ARTERITIS

From ten to fifty percent of people with PMR have detectable giant-cell arteritis. Scientists do not fully understand the relationship between these two diseases. In giant-cell arteritis, certain arteries (large blood vessels) in the body become inflamed. The inflammation occurs in the walls of the arteries and damages the elastic fibers found there. The term "giant cell" describes the large cells containing several nuclei characteristically found in the vessel walls. Inflammation causes the arteries to become narrow, and sometimes completely blocks some of the arteries. Severe giant-cell arteritis can lead to loss of blood flow to a vital organ, resulting in loss of vision, a stroke, or a heart attack.

For these reasons, people with PMR should be aware of the warning signs of giant-cell arteritis (sometimes called temporal arteritis) and report any of them immediately to their doctors. One symptom is pain, swelling, redness, and heat in the area of the blood vessels on the upper front sides of the head, near the temples. These vessels are called the temporal arteries. With inflammation, they may become enlarged and painful, and the area may be tender to the touch. Headaches commonly occur. Other symptoms suggesting giant-cell arteritis of the temporal arteries include changes in vision, such as seeing double, blurring, or blind spots. Since the disease can cause blindness, any problems with one's vision should be reported at once to the physician. Pain in the jaw when chewing; dizziness; or hearing trouble can be other warning signals of temporal arteritis.

The diagnosis of temporal arteritis is made by removing a small bit of one of the temporal arteries through an incision in the scalp. If the disease is present when the biopsied tissue is examined with a microscope, the artery will contain damaged elastic fibers and show typical signs of inflammation, usually with giant cells.

The treatment of temporal arteritis must be begun immediately with a large dose of prednisone or another corticosteroid. Large doses of these drugs are used to avoid the danger of blindness from damage to the artery that nourishes the optic nerve. If started early enough, corticosteroid treatment is successful.

THE FUTURE

Fortunately, both PMR and giant-cell arteritis usually go away on their own. However, it is difficult to tell how long either will last, since the duration of both conditions is different from person to person.

Eventually, most people with PMR can also expect that the dosage of medication they take will be gradually reduced and eventually stopped altogether. In the meantime, people with PMR can lead normal lives with only minor adjustments in their daily routines. They must, however, continue to watch for flare-ups of their disease, for symptoms of giant-cell arteritis, and for side effects of their drugs, and must continue to see their doctors regularly.

CHAPTER TWENTY-THREE

Fibrositis

At one time or another, everyone has had temporary aches and pains in various parts of the body. These symptoms may be caused by the flu, from overusing a limb, or from sitting in a hunched position while reading or watching TV. A person may wake up stiff in the morning perhaps as a result of sleeping in an awkward position.

Such pains are seldom troublesome and soon disappear by themselves, but when pain, stiffness, and aching become constant, most people go to a doctor to find out what is causing such discomfort. It may be fibrositis. Although the word may be strange, fibrositis is a common ailment.

Doctors have still not agreed on what causes fibrositis, how to diagnose it, and how to treat it. Although the word "fibrositis" literally means inflammation of fibrous connective tissue, there is no inflammation present. Many physicians believe that fibrositis is so poorly defined that they do not ever make this diagnosis.

Nonetheless there are many people with chronic pain in the muscles, tendons, and about the joints who do not have a true arthritis or another cause of pain that can be identified by any medical testing or examination. Some physicians use different names to describe such conditions:

- Musculoskeletal pain syndrome

- Nonarticular rheumatism ("non" = not, "artic" = joint)

- Muscular rheumatism
- Fibromyalgia ("my" = muscle, "algia" = pain)

Doctors have no general agreement about the use of these terms. Whatever they may be called, however, their symptoms are very real. In the last few years more physicians have become interested in these conditions because they are so common and produce so much pain. Some people clearly do not fall into a single category that can be called fibrositis.

In most kinds of arthritis, disease of the joints causes pain and swelling that can lead to damage and crippling. But in fibrositis the pain is in the ligaments, tendons, and muscles. Since the pain of fibrositis may worsen after moving a joint, people with fibrositis often think that joint disease is causing their pain.

Yet, because fibrositis does not actually damage the joints, it will never cause deformity or crippling. It is not an inherited disorder, so there is no need to worry about passing it on to the next generation.

More often than not, symptoms eventually go away by themselves. In the meantime, the disease can last for months, or years. Doctors have no way to predict how long the symptoms may last in a given individual. Most people, however, can keep their symptoms under control by following the treatment programs that they have worked out in cooperation with their doctors.

AFFECTED POPULATION

Anyone can get fibrositis. However, more women than men have fibrositis, and most of the people affected are between the ages of thirty-five and sixty. Fibrositis tends to affect women approaching the age of menopause more often than at other times. Fibrositis can also occur as a manifestation of rheumatoid arthritis, ankylosing spondylitis, and other rheumatic diseases.

PHYSICAL EFFECTS

Some of the pain of fibrositis may be due to tense muscles. You can demonstrate the effect of the disease for yourself with

229

a simple experiment. If you clench your fist tightly and keep it that way, within about a minute you'll feel a burning pain beginning to spread up your arm. This is the pain of muscle contraction, which can contribute to the pain felt in fibrositis.

The primary symptom of fibrositis is pain. Most people feel the pain of fibrositis as aching, stiffness, and tenderness around joints, muscles, tendons, and ligaments. The pain may appear in various areas of the body, but tends to be worst around the shoulders, in the back, and around the hips. People with fibrositis usually sleep poorly and often don't feel rested when they wake up in the morning. One study showed that electroencephalograms (brain wave patterns) taken of people with fibrositis while they slept did not register the typical "deep sleep" pattern characteristic of people without fibrositis. In another study, volunteer students without symptoms who were kept awake all night by ringing or a buzzer whenever they fell asleep developed pain and soreness in muscles very similar to those of fibrositis.

The symptoms of fibrositis are usually present when the person first wakes up, but the discomfort usually increases as the day goes on and the person becomes more active. Physical and emotional fatigue are often present. Feelings of anxiety and depression can make the person feel even more helpless in tolerating the pain, making it seem worse than ever.

DIAGNOSIS

Fibrositis is difficult to diagnose because no specific laboratory test can detect it. In fact, normal tests may lead the doctor to suspect fibrositis as the cause of the pain.

An extremely important part of the diagnostic process is the person's full description and explanation of the symptoms. The description should include the times of day the pain is worse and the activities, such as housework, typing, studying, or sports, that increase the pain. Because symptoms of fibrositis are often made worse by emotional stress, it is important to be frank and open with your doctor in telling him or her about any situation in your life that is causing concern or frustration. This may involve your relationship with your spouse or other people who are close to you, problems with your job, your sexual life, financial worries, or other concerns. Unless your doctor knows all about these matters, he or she cannot treat you successfully.

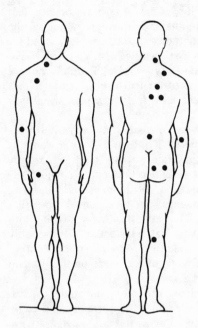

Trigger spots in fibrositis

On physical examination the doctor will find certain highly tender spots (trigger points) over the muscles in the back of the neck and shoulders, the side of the breastbone, the buttocks, and the sides of the knees and elbows.

The physician will also examine the arms, legs, and spine to see if movement of these parts causes pain. In fibrositis, certain muscles may be tender when squeezed, especially around the lower back and buttocks.

POSSIBLE CAUSES

No one yet knows the causes of fibrositis. The same symptoms of fibrositis are often present in many other diseases, including other rheumatic diseases, blood diseases, cancers, infections, hormonal problems, and reactions to drugs. When the symptoms are caused by or accompany another disease, the condition is called secondary fibrositis.

Since emotional factors often have a significant role in

231

bringing on attacks of fibrositis, some physicians believe that fibrositis is a psychosomatic illness. However, studies of the personalities and emotional characteristics of people with fibrositis have not demonstrated that people with fibrositis have more emotional problems than anyone else. People who are tense or anxious, who have pent-up frustrations and feelings of hostility, or who feel depressed do feel more pain from their fibrositis.

Because laboratory tests have failed to show any abnormalities, some people have wondered if individuals with fibrositis are suffering from actual pain. Pain coming from apparently normal muscles and tendons is difficult to comprehend. Perhaps comparing it with a headache will help in understanding fibrositis. Everyone has headaches, and everyone knows that the pain they cause is real. But almost always, X-rays and other tests done on someone who has a headache will probably give normal results. Yet for unknown reasons, normal structures like the muscles in the back of the neck or the arteries that lead to the head are causing pain.

The same is true in fibrositis. Apparently normal muscles, tendons, and ligaments somehow behave abnormally and cause pain. Why? The tender trigger points that are nearly always present have led some to suspect that an abnormal sensitivity to pain may be an underlying cause of fibrositis. Perhaps stimuli such as normal joint motion that cause no pain in most people can irritate hypersensitive nerve endings in people with fibrositis. However, one study has shown that although people with this condition have abnormal pain sensitivity over trigger point areas, their pain sensation in other parts of the body is perfectly normal.

TREATMENT

Unfortunately, there is no cure for fibrositis. With the doctor's guidance, the person who has this condition must try to keep the symptoms under control so that he or she can lead a normal life without much pain. A typical treatment program for persons with fibrositis includes medication; physical therapy, special exercises or both; and the use of heat or cold to relieve pain. The affected individual may need some help in recognizing or solving emotional problems that could create tension and aggravate the condition.

Medication

Aspirin and the other nonsteroidal drugs can usually relieve the pain of fibrositis to some extent but are seldom completely successful. It may be necessary to try several of these drugs in succession before finding one that works. The sleep disturbance which is such a common part of fibrositis may be helped by a group of drugs called tricyclic anti-depressants. The most widely used one, amitriptyline, is usually given as a single dose at bedtime. Sometimes sedatives taken at bedtime or in small doses during the day may be helpful.

Because there is no inflammation in fibrositis, corticosteroids or the long-lasting drugs used in rheumatoid arthritis are of no value. Besides prescribing drugs taken by mouth, doctors sometimes inject a muscle-relaxing drug or a local anesthetic directly into a painful area to bring about muscle relaxation more quickly.

Physical Therapy

Physical therapy can help the person with fibrositis to relax tense muscles; it can range from formal sessions with a physical therapist to simple exercises done at home.

Besides teaching muscle relaxation, physical therapy can also help persons with fibrositis to learn to change their postures. Poor posture can make the condition worse. The physical therapist will also show the person how to use heat or cold to relax muscles and reduce pain. This treatment may involve warm baths, showers, hot packs, and heating pads. Sometimes therapists give ultrasound treatment or massage the muscles with mechanical vibrators.

Some people with fibrositis benefit from one or more relaxation techniques, including body awareness programs, transcendental meditation, biofeedback, and relaxation tapes. All of these methods teach control and relaxation of the muscles. Transcutaneous electrical stimulation, a technique in which low-voltage electrical current is passed through the skin, is sometimes of value but its effects tend to wear off after a month or two. Anyone considering such a program should first consult his or her doctor or physical therapist to be certain of its potential benefits.

Changing the Environment

Changing certain daily habits may make a difference for the person with fibrositis. For example, pain in the neck, arms, and shoulders can be brought on by long hours of typing. If this is the case, it is usually possible to relieve the pain simply by raising the height of the typewriter. A firmer mattress may help prevent morning stiffness. Some people find a water bed beneficial. If driving in heavy traffic makes the muscles tighten up and the problem is not solved by adjusting the sitting position behind the wheel, then other forms of transportation, such as car pools or buses, may be the answer.

Emotional Factors

People with fibrositis need to pay attention to their emotions. Feelings are harder to pin down and understand than physical symptoms, but some people are unable to make real progress in overcoming fibrositis until some basic emotional problem is brought into the open and resolved.

Emotional distress can be handled in a variety of ways. A few sessions with a sympathetic doctor or counselor may be all that is needed. Sessions in which the doctor meets with the entire family may help someone with fibrositis deal with stress and better understand their other feelings. Some people may need psychiatric evaluation and therapy in order to discuss their hidden feelings or real situations that may be making them worse. Others may have a depression that can be treated successfully with certain drugs. Help with the emotional aspects of life may be a very important part of the treatment program for fibrositis.

THE FUTURE

The vast majority of people with fibrositis can and should continue their usual activities. They may have to modify some aspects of their lives, and may even add some new activities to their daily routines, such as yoga classes or set periods for practicing relaxation techniques. The disease will flare up from time to time. When an approaching flare-up is felt, the doctor should be asked how to handle it.

On the other hand, because fibrositis is frequently self-limiting, it may eventually disappear permanently with a regular program of treatment designed for the particular situation of the person who has it. With practice, it is possible to learn to control the body, relax the muscles, and avoid the pain of fibrositis. They can also learn to recognize activities or situations that can cause their pain to become worse. Most people with the condition don't know how to relax and must learn to do so. When this goal is reached, they will be able to control the disease instead of letting it control them.

CHAPTER TWENTY-FOUR

Bursitis, Tendonitis and the Painful Shoulder

Bursitis and tendonitis are rheumatic conditions. Bursitis means pain due to inflammation in a bursa, a small sac of fluid which acts as a cushion between a tendon and a bone. Tendonitis means painful inflammation or irritation of a tendon, the band of tissue similar to a rope, that connects a muscle to a bone. Both of these structures are illustrated in Chapter 2. Bursitis and tendonitis differ from most of the other diseases in important ways:

- In tendonitis and bursitis, inflammation involves the parts that surround the joint instead of the joint itself.

- Bursitis and tendonitis usually affect only one isolated part of the body at a time, instead of several joints.

- Bursitis and tendonitis often result from a specific activity or injury, unlike most rheumatic diseases, which usually arise without any obvious cause.

- Many forms of arthritis are chronic and disabling. Bursitis and tendonitis usually, though not always, last only a short time and often go away without causing permanent damage.

AFFECTED POPULATION
AND POSSIBLE CAUSES

Bursitis and tendonitis occur most often in people over thirty. Exceptions are people who have been very active in sports or whose work calls for the same movement over and over. The wear and tear of repeated use takes its toll on bursae and tendons, just as it does on other parts of the body. Most adults have experienced some of these changes in the tissues around their joints.

With enough stress on a joint or tendon, anyone can develop bursitis or tendonitis. For example, they can occur in someone who is not used to a certain kind of exercise and suddenly has an extensive workout. A sudden stress, like jerking up a heavy package, can also lead to tendonitis.

PHYSICAL EFFECTS

An episode of bursitis or tendonitis can occur in many different parts of the body. The most common area affected by bursitis is the shoulder. Other regions of the body that may be affected by bursitis or tendonitis include the hip, the elbow, the knees, the Achilles tendon in the heel, the wrists, fingers, and the ankles.

Both conditions often begin suddenly, and almost all episodes of both improve within days or weeks. If treated correctly, either condition rarely causes lasting pains or loss of function. Some people have repeated attacks, usually in the same part of the body or in another region.

The primary symptom of bursitis or tendonitis is pain. The pain may be so severe that the person cannot move the affected part. The pain of bursitis or tendonitis often awakens people at night, when it begins and interferes with their sleep.

Since bursae and tendons usually are situated very close to each other, it is not always possible to distinguish between bursitis and tendonitis. Some of the common types of both are described here according to where they occur in the body.

Shoulder

The shoulder is a complex joint because it can be moved in so many different directions. Its function depends on the proper alignment and operation of several groups of muscles and tendons, and it is subject to many different types of injury. The muscles of the shoulder (deltoid and rotator cuff muscles) and upper arm all unite to cover the upper end of the upper arm bone (which is known as the humerus). The rotator cuff is made up of the tendons of five muscles which rotate the arm both inward and outward. A bursa lies between these tendons and muscles, acting as a cushion. The tendons and the bursa lie between two bony surfaces—the head of the humerus and a part of the shoulder bone, or scapula, called the acromion. Some of the problems that can occur in the shoulder area include the painful shoulder syndrome (acute subdeltoid bursitis), the shoulder-hand syndrome, and bicipital tendonitis.

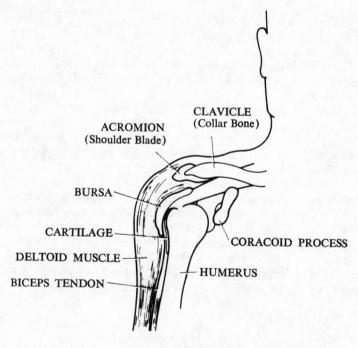

Shoulder anatomy

Painful Shoulder Syndrome (Acute Subdeltoid Bursitis)

By moving the arm in the wrong way, a person can pinch one or more of the tendons, catching them between two bony surfaces. The result may be irritated, inflamed tendons. Sometimes the tendons become inflamed without being pinched. When the tendons become inflamed, the bursa next to them can also become inflamed.

An acute attack of the painful shoulder syndrome usually comes on suddenly within a few hours and is excruciatingly painful. The tendons may be so painful and swollen that they can't move under the overhanging bone. When that happens, it becomes impossible to bring the arm up from the side or to rotate it in either direction. The only movement that can be made will come from the shoulder blade alone, since the shoulder joint can't move. Combing the hair or reaching back to put a coat on is painful. Fortunately, it often goes away in a few days with treatment, though it may recur at a later date. If it doesn't go away, proper medical treatment will usually be successful.

Shoulder-Hand Syndrome

There are many theories about the cause of the shoulder-hand syndrome, but it usually starts with irritation of the nerves in the shoulder. This irritation triggers a nerve response in the spinal cord that results in nerve impulses being transmitted to the blood vessels, sweat glands, and hair follicles of the hand.

The shoulder symptoms of the shoulder-hand syndrome include pain and limited arm movement. The hand symptoms begin with weakness and stiffness, so that the affected person cannot make a full fist. The hand may feel as if it is being burned. It will be extremely sensitive to the slightest touch. Even the touch of a bed sheet may be painful. The hand and the fingers usually swell, and the hand will feel cold and moist. The skin color may turn bluish-white.

The swelling and pain may gradually go away even without treatment. However, by the time they do the muscles of the hand may have wasted away, and the joints may have stiffened. Eventually, the hand can become deformed and the fingers immobilized.

Fortunately, permanent damage can usually be prevented

by early diagnosis and treatment of the shoulder-hand syndrome. Anyone who has severe shoulder and hand pain that persists for more than a week should see a doctor at once, so that treatment can be started. Sometimes the shoulder-hand syndrome may develop as part of some other condition, such as a stroke, heart attack, pleurisy (fluid in the lungs), or after a blow to the shoulder or the hand. Usually no obvious cause can be found, but the syndrome tends to occur in women under severe emotional stress. Helping the person manage whatever stress she is under is an important part of successful treatment in such cases.

Bicipital Tendonitis

This condition is usually due to a small tear of the tendon that attaches the biceps muscle to the shoulder bone (scapula). Pain is most severe during heavy lifting or strenuous activity.

Other Shoulder Problems

Although they are not examples of bursitis or tendonitis, three other types of shoulder problems deserve mention: cuff tear, damage to the acromioclavicular joint, and frozen shoulder.

A cuff tear is a tear or split of one or more of the tendons that are attached to the rotator cuff. The tear can be partial or complete. A partial cuff tear causes considerable pain that may last a long time. The person has difficulty raising the arm above a horizontal position. Partial tears of the cuff tendons usually heal by themselves if the arm is kept in a sling for some time and then gradually exercised.

With a complete cuff tear it becomes impossible even to bring the arm out from the side without help from the other arm or from another person. To decide whether such a problem is due to a complete cuff tear or to extreme pain from a partial tear, the physician may inject a local anesthetic into the arm and ask the affected person to try the motion again. A tear can be diagnosed by injection of a dye into the shoulder, a procedure called an arthrogram. If a complete tear is the diagnosis, surgery may be needed to close it. The results are usually very good.

Sometimes shoulder pain is caused by arthritis in the acromioclavicular joint. This joint is at the tip of the shoulder, where the end of the collar bone, or clavicle, meets the acromion, or outer point of the shoulder blade.

When this joint is affected, any arm movement causes pain in the tip of the shoulder, but particularly shrugging of the shoulders.

Frozen shoulder occurs for reasons that are poorly understood. More women are affected by this disorder than men. The capsule, or lining, of the shoulder joint shrinks as a result of the growth of scar tissue in it. As a result, the shoulder becomes painful and the person has difficulty moving the shoulder over a period of weeks to months. Diagnosis can be aided by an arthrogram.

Elbow

Tennis Elbow

This term is used to describe inflammation of the bony prominence at the outer side of the elbow. Tennis elbow does not happen only in tennis players. A frequent cause is a sudden tightening of some of the muscles in the hand and forearm, such as occurs when throwing something heavy or taking a backhand swing in tennis. Most often the problem is caused by repeated motions involving the elbow. The person with tennis elbow has most pain when straightening the elbow against resistance, as when hitting a backhand shot in tennis. Lifting may be painful and the outside of the elbow may be tender. However, the elbow motion itself remains normal or close to normal.

Hand

"Trigger Finger"

This condition is caused by an inflammation of the tendons used in bending the fingers. One cause may be a sudden blow or other trauma to the fingers. Bumps form on the tendons and become trapped within the outer tendon lining, blocking the motion of the fingers and causing pain.

DeQuervain's Wrist

In most people who have this condition, it is related to repeated use of or trauma to the wrist. Tendons in the wrist, particularly the one which extends the thumb, become painful and sometimes swollen. Pain comes with the use of the thumb or wrist, as using pruning shears, knitting, or writing for long periods. Avoiding the activities that cause the problem usually helps to relieve the pain.

Hip

Trochanteric Bursitis

In this type of bursitis, which can be very painful, a bursa near the hip joint becomes inflamed. The bursa is located in the side of the upper thigh over a bony protuberance called the greater trochanter. The pain is made worse by climbing, sitting for a prolonged period, or sleeping on the affected side of the body. The inflammation may be caused by a difference in the lengths of the legs, and if so, usually occurs on the side of the longer leg. However, in most people, the cause of trochanteric bursitis is not known.

"Tailor's Seat"

This condition, also known as "weaver's bottom," refers to an inflammation in the bursa over the ischium (the lower part of the hip bone in the buttocks). It can be extremely painful, and is made worse by sitting, especially on a hard surface. It is one of the few conditions that cause more pain when sitting than when standing.

Knee

"Housemaid's Knee"

This disorder is an inflammation of the bursa just in front of the kneecap. The front of the knee feels tender, usually because of repeated irritation to the affected part of the joint from frequent kneeling.

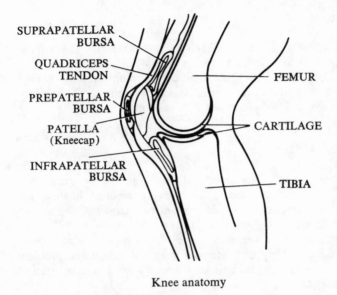

Knee anatomy

"Clergyman's Knee"

The effect of this condition is similar to that of housemaid's knee, except the bursitis occurs just below the knee bone.

Injury and Inflammation of the Tendons in the Knee

Tendonitis of the knee is fairly common in growing children. A failure to warm-up correctly before participating in sports activities may also cause injury to the tendons.

Anserine Bursitis

Three of the thigh muscles attach to the top of one of the long bones in the lower leg. These three muscles have a common tendon, the anserine tendon, under which is a bursa. Inflammation of this bursa can lead to pain and tenderness on the inside of the knee. Usually, the knee itself is not painful to move.

Ankle

A common form of tendonitis of the ankle may result from an injury to the Achilles tendon, particularly if the tendon is torn. The person with this condition commonly reports having heard a snapping noise when the injury occurred. This injury is quite painful and can result in loss of motion of the ankle.

DIAGNOSIS

The doctor has three basic tools to use in making a diagnosis of bursitis or tendonitis. They are the medical history, the results of a physical examination, and sometimes X-rays.

The answers to a series of questions by the doctor will show whether someone's recent activities could have caused bursitis or tendonitis. They also help the doctor decide if the problem is a local attack of bursitis or tendonitis or a sign of a more general condition.

The physical examination provides additional information on the source of the pain. The doctor will identify the most painful area by palpating. He or she will also test your ability to carry out certain motions in order to pinpoint what structures are involved and if there are any serious tears of tendons or ligaments. Although few laboratory tests can confirm the presence of bursitis or tendonitis, certain tests can be done to rule out other diseases.

X-rays are sometimes used in order to be certain that no other conditions are contributing to the problem. They will sometimes show the presence of calcium deposits, which can help in making a diagnosis of bursitis, especially in the shoulder. Arthrograms may be done for some suspected problems such as a frozen shoulder or a torn rotator cuff. A special dye is injected that allows subsequent X-rays to visualize the soft tissue such as tendons which do not show up on ordinary X-rays.

TREATMENT

Once the doctor is sure that a person has bursitis, tendonitis, or both, a treatment program will be planned. Since each person's situation is different, the treatment program is individually tailored, taking into consideration the specific diagnosis, the severity of the problem, and the person's age, occupation, and favorite sports or other activities.

Early Phase Treatment

For some people with bursitis, tendonitis, or both, such as those with the painful shoulder syndrome, a rest period will be prescribed. Other common measures for the early treatment of a painful shoulder include putting the arm in a sling for rest and protection. The arm will be bent at the elbow and held against the body. The person may also be told to apply ice to the painful area of the arm three or four times a day, using ice packs or towels filled with ice cubes for periods of twenty minutes at a time.

Exercise

After the painful part of the body begins to improve, it must slowly begin to be exercised again, so as to prevent the loss of motion in the joint. The doctor or physical therapist may demonstrate how to do special exercises at home. They may also explain ways to avoid straining the affected area. Sometimes a person may need to see a physical therapist or occupational therapist several times a week to receive treatment.

Part of the treatment for bursitis or tendonitis may include changing some daily activities, or even giving up a few. Usually, a person's activities can be modified so that his or her lifestyle doesn't change dramatically.

Even when normal motion again becomes possible, the person with bursitis or tendonitis may still have some pain. If the exercise program is followed as directed, the pain will eventually go away.

Medication

The doctor will probably prescribe medication to relieve the pain of bursitis or tendonitis, and to reduce the inflammation that causes the pain. The most commonly used drugs for both conditions are aspirin, nonsteroidal anti-inflammatory drugs, corticosteroid drugs, and anesthetics.

The corticosteroids are not usually taken by mouth to treat bursitis and tendonitis. However, they are often injected directly into bursae in acute situations. When they are used in this way, their potentially dangerous side effects can be minimized. Large doses of a steroid given by mouth are often used to treat the shoulder-hand syndrome. If so, the doctor will closely watch the person taking the drug to keep the side effects to a minimum.

An anesthetic such as xylocaine may be used to produce a nerve block in treating the shoulder-hand syndrome. The anesthetic is injected into small nerve bodies (sympathetic ganglia) in the neck next to the spine. This treatment is aimed at stopping the nerve irritation that accompanies the syndrome. These injections may be needed for two to six weeks. Sometimes the injections work only temporarily, and the symptoms return. Rarely, a person may need to have the sympathetic ganglia removed surgically.

Heat and Other Treatments

When ice is used initially for very acute pain and inflammation, the doctor may recommend that the ice treatment be replaced with heat treatment after the first forty-eight hours. The heat can be applied with hot packs, a heating pad, an infrared lamp, or hot showers. The doctor or physical therapist can recommend the best method for a particular situation.

For someone with a severe hand problem, such as shoulder-hand syndrome, the doctor and physical therapist may try other kinds of treatment. Electrical stimulation may be used to make the muscles contract and help the person learn to contract them on his or her own. Biofeedback is another technique for teaching someone to regain control over muscle movement. A nerve block can be used on the nerves that go from the spinal cord to the affected muscles as another means of bringing a damaged hand back to normal.

Surgery

Surgery is rarely necessary for the treatment of bursitis or tendonitis. It may be needed, however, to repair a complete cuff tear or to remove calcium deposits from an acutely painful shoulder. In some people with a cuff tear, an operation to fuse or permanently join the shoulder joint may be required. People with very severe damage to the acromioclavicular joint may benefit from an operation to repair the joint and reduce the pain.

THE FUTURE

A person who has had one attack of bursitis or tendonitis will not necessarily have similar, later episodes. Even someone who has had two or three acute attacks can avoid having more of them in the future by eliminating or reducing those activities known to have originally caused the problem. The best way to prevent attacks of bursitis or tendonitis is to stay with a planned exercise program until the doctor or therapist advises stopping it. This will build up muscle strength, and full range of motion of the sore joint should eventually return; both improvements will help prevent future problems.

CHAPTER TWENTY-FIVE

Back Pain and Arthritis

Back pain is one of the most common health problems in the United States. Some studies have shown that as many as fifty to eighty percent of adults in Western countries have had such pain at some time. In the United States, back pain is a leading cause of time lost from work, and costs about fourteen billion dollars each year for treatment and disability payments.

Pain in the back can range from an uncomfortable ache to a severe and agonizing spasm. It can last for a day or two, or it can continue for weeks, months, or years. Besides injury or disease, back pain has been blamed on a host of problems including emotional upsets, poor posture, lack of exercise, and obesity

Back pain is part of many of the one hundred or more kinds of rheumatic diseases. As a result, rheumatologists and other health professionals with a special interest in arthritis frequently care for people with back pain.

More often, however, back pain occurs for reasons other than a rheumatic disease. It can be brought on by injury, poor muscle tone, physical stress such as from lifting a heavy object incorrectly, or environmental stress such as from sitting all day in a chair of the wrong height. Back pain can also be part of such conditions as tumors, infections, or abnormalities in body chemistry. Unfortunately, in the majority of cases of persistent back pain the cause cannot be determined.

AFFECTED POPULATION

Every year, more than three percent of the American population have a back pain problem severe enough to require a doctor's attention. Although back pain can appear at any age, most people are first affected between the ages of thirty and forty. Men are more likely to have back pain early in life. But starting in middle age, the problem begins to affect more women than men. Among people with arthritis, back pain occurs most often in those whose knees, hips, and spine are involved.

PHYSICAL EFFECTS

Before reading further about the causes and different kinds of back pain, you may find it helpful to review the description of the structure of the back as described in Chapter 15. Back pain can result from disease or injury to any of the structures in the back: the ligaments supporting the spine, the vertebrae, the pelvic bone, the ribs, the joints connecting the vertebrae, the nerves emerging from the spinal cord, the spinal cord itself, and the connective tissue surrounding the muscles that move the spine.

Nearly everyone has had a brief spell of back pain at one time or another. These twinges are usually spasms, or uncontrolled contractions, of the muscles of the back. They may be caused by sudden movements such as turning around quickly or bending down to pick something up, particularly when a twisting motion is also involved. The twinges usually disappear rapidly of their own accord, and don't require a doctor's care. Some people develop acute, or short-term, back pain. This pain can appear suddenly or come on gradually over a period of hours or days. It may be felt only in the back or may spread to the arms or legs. This is the kind of back pain for which most people seek a doctor's help. In some people, the pain is a mild one that simply will not go away within a few days or a week. Others have a pain they describe as unbearable, as if they were tied in a knot. With this kind of pain, they have trouble finding any position that is comfortable.

A few people experience chronic, or long-term, back pain that lasts for more than three or four weeks. There are many possible causes of this chronic pain.

POSSIBLE CAUSES

Anything that puts pressure or tension on the nerves in the back and surrounding structures can cause pain. For example, obesity adds to the load the back already carries, and overtaxes the muscles that hold it up. Therefore a minor stress to the back that would not affect the average person could be painful to a person who is overweight. People with poor posture may put extra stress on back muscles and joints by making a few of them do all the work. Also, people who don't get enough exercise are more prone to get sore backs because the support muscles don't have enough strength and tire easily.

Injuries often cause back pain. Along with accidents and sports injuries, back problems can result simply from the improper performance of such routine activities as lifting, turning, or bending. When done the wrong way, for example, lifting a heavy object without bending the knees, these actions can strain muscles and ligaments in the back and damage the cartilage discs between the vertebrae.

As mentioned, back pain is also a symptom of some kinds of arthritis. One such condition is ankylosing spondylitis, a chronic disease that causes inflammation and stiffness of the intervertebral joints. Ligaments near these joints are sacroiliac and primary sites of inflammation. Back pain may also be caused by osteoarthritis, which results in a breakdown of the cartilage that cushions the joints. This condition may affect the intervertebral joints directly or cause back pain indirectly when it occurs in other joints, such as the hips or knees, where bony spurs usually develop and lead to back problems. Back pain may also occur in people with rheumatoid arthritis, polymyalgia rheumatica, fibrositis, and other less common rheumatic diseases.

Tension and emotional upsets can lead to or aggravate back pain. Mental stress, fatigue, and too much worry can cause the back muscles to tighten and go into a spasm. Tension can make an existing back condition worsen. If the cause of stress can be identified and relieved, the pain may improve.

A few people get back pain as the result of underlying diseases or structural problems in the spine. This small group includes people with "slipped" discs—which do not really slip out of location, but rather bulge out so that they press against the nerves branching out from the spinal cord. The pressure on these nerves is what causes the back pain in this condition. Other people may have back pain caused by an infection in the bones or joints of the back, a tumor, abnormal curvature of the spine (scoliosis), or a bone-thinning disease called osteoporosis. Osteoporosis is most common in women past their menopause and in people who take corticosteroid drugs for a long period. Certain types of kidney problems, diseases affecting the female reproductive organs, and conditions involving the lining of the lung (pleura) may cause back pain.

DIAGNOSIS

As in making any diagnosis, the doctor begins an examination for the cause of back pain by asking about the details of the symptoms. He or she may ask many questions, such as where the pain is strongest, what might have set it off, whether other family members have similar complaints (especially if ankylosing spondylitis is suspected, since it sometimes runs in families), whether an emotional upset or stress helped cause the pain, what other health problems also exist, and the relationship of the pain to any related or other activities. If the pain is made worse by coughing, it is probably due to a herniated disc. If the affected person is a woman, is over sixty and has had her ovaries removed when she was thirty, she probably has osteoporosis.

The doctor will also perform a physical examination, paying close attention to the muscles and joints that may be involved in the pain. The affected person will be asked to perform many different motions while the doctor checks for problems in muscle contraction or in the ligaments, tendons, or other tissues. The doctor will also see if the person has areas of tenderness that suggest damage to internal organs such as the kidneys, the intestines, or other organs. He or she may also measure the person's chest expansion to see whether the joints that attach the ribs to the vertebrae are affected by ankylosing spondylitis. Careful testings of the muscle strength, skin sensation (usually with a pin), and tendon reflexes in the legs are important elements of the physical examination, because the nerves to the legs all pass out of the spinal canal and down the back of the legs. Many conditions causing back pain can interfere with the nerve supply to the legs.

After the physical examination, the doctor will usually decide to do special tests. Occasionally, X-rays show the cause of back pain, although they are usually not very helpful. X-rays will indicate whether a person has a fractured vertebra; a form of arthritis such as osteoarthritis or ankylosing spondylitis; bony growths on the vertebrae (hyperostosis); a vertebra that has slipped forward (spondylolisthesis); infections of a disc or bones; a tumor; or a deformity in bone structure.

Certain conditions, particularly those which cause pressure on nerve roots or the spinal cord, can also be shown with computerized axial tomography, or a "CAT" scan. This kind of scan gives the doctor a three-dimensional view of the body, and can reveal problems that may not show up on X-rays. However, it is only needed for a small percentage of people who have back pain.

Another test that may be done for back pain is a myelogram, in which a special dye is injected into the spinal canal, allowing disc abnormalities to show up on X-rays. Because bulging discs cannot be seen on ordinary X-rays, a myelogram helps the doctor make this diagnosis and identify the location of a disc rupture that requires surgery.

Blood tests are not very helpful in diagnosing the causes of back pain. One test that may be done is the erythrocyte sedimentation rate. If an inflammatory illness such as ankylosing spondylitis is causing the pain, the sedimentation rate will usually be higher than normal.

After taking a complete medical history, performing a careful physical examination, and studying the results of X-rays and laboratory tests, the physician may still not be able to make a precise diagnosis of the cause of chronic back pain. Sometimes a person with a back pain complaint may be malingering (pretending to have pain that is not actually present). An experienced physician can usually tell when a person is not telling the truth. More often, the pain is real, but the examination and tests yield normal results. Emotional and psychological factors may sometimes cause such pain or make it worse. However, medical science still has much to learn about lower back pain. More sensitive instruments and techniques are needed to detect and measure changes in the structure and tissues of the back in people with unexplained back pain before the answers can be found.

TREATMENT

Once the cause or causes of back pain have been identified as closely as possible, a treatment program will be designed to specifically ease the problem causing it. The program may include a combination of rest, heat and cold treatments, posture training, special exercises, and medication.

Rest

Often, the first treatment the doctor will prescribe for back pain is rest. The amount of rest needed will differ from one person to another. Some people, especially those with disc disease, may need to spend time in a hospital for specialized care. Alternatively, bed rest at home with a board between the mattress and box spring of a person's bed may be adequate. Even if bed rest is not needed, a temporary back support may be necessary to help take the stress off the painful area. Special devices or pillows may be suggested to support the neck, middle of the back, or feet.

Heat and Cold

Hot and cold treatments often help relieve back pain. Heat relaxes tight muscles, and the numbing effect of cold helps to ease pain. The doctor, nurse, or therapist can suggest appropriate heat- and cold-treatment methods for specific problems.

Posture and Shoes

For some people, posture training and exercise help relieve back pain. It is possible to easily learn better ways of lifting, bending over, and carrying objects by keeping the back in a normal position and using the legs as much as possible when bending. The person with back pain should also try to distribute any load he or she lifts across as many muscles and joints as possible. For example, both arms should be used instead of one, and it is possible to slide many objects rather than carry them.

253

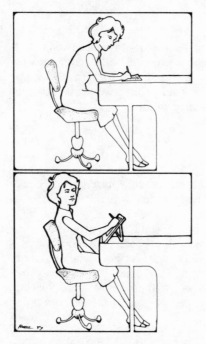

Correct vs. incorrect sitting positions for the person with back pain

Whether a person is lying down, sitting, standing, walking, or lifting, the back should be kept straight. This habit helps to avoid putting too much stress on any group of muscles or joints. Using a firm mattress or a board between the mattress and box spring of the bed will help to maintain correct posture during sleep or resting in bed. Changes in sitting posture are especially important for people who sit at work or home for long periods, and such people should be sure to avoid slumping.

An occupational or physical therapist can help analyze and correct problems with posture, movements, lifting and carrying objects, and work-related physical tasks. These professionals may be able to help pinpoint the cause of the pain and suggest helpful exercises or different ways of performing certain tasks. They may also recommend new forms of recreation or different ways for the person to continue his or her daily activities.

Footwear is another important part of posture. High heels can put more stress on the lower back than low or flat heels do. Shoes should be strong enough to provide support for the feet and prevent the legs from tiring.

Exercise and Weight Loss

For many people, the key to a healthy back is maintaining a regular exercise program. Some exercises improve posture; others help strengthen the muscles that support the back. The right kind of exercise program can do a lot to keep a back problem under control and permit the continuation of regular activities. Doctors and therapists can help each person plan the right kind of exercise.

One exercise that helps people improve their posture and often relieves low back pain is called the pelvic tilt. It is done by lying on one's back on the floor with the knees bent and feet flat. With the hands resting on the stomach, the lower back is pressed against the floor by pulling in the stomach and tightening the buttocks. With practice, it will become possible to hold this position when walking or standing.

Although being overweight may not itself cause back pain, it does add to the load the back has to carry, since it leads to a stretching of certain muscles that support the back. Since being overweight can also make other health problems more serious, the doctor may recommend weight loss as one way of reducing back pain and improving one's general health. People with back pain should ask their doctors to recommend a nutritionally balanced weight-loss diet. A fad diet can be harmful if necessary nutrients are left out, and may cause new problems instead of solving old ones.

Both weight loss and exercise programs should be supervised by a doctor or other qualified health professional. As with diet, the wrong kind of exercise can be harmful.

Other Physical Treatments

Learning relaxation exercises or participating in biofeedback training are often useful ways of helping the back muscles to relax, and of reducing pain. Psychologists and other health

255

professionals who have training in the use of these techniques can help the person with back pain to learn them. Such people should discuss with their doctors the question of whether such training may benefit them.

Medication

Medication to relieve the pain, relax tight muscles, or reduce inflammation can be an important addition to the treatment program though it seldom relieves the symptoms by itself. The medication needed depends on the kind of back pain that exists. Different medications are available for acute pain, chronic pain, pain brought on by an injury, and pain that is related to emotional stress.

For some people whose back pain is caused by a rheumatic disease, doctors give medications that reduce inflammation and relieve pain. These include aspirin or other nonsteroidal anti-inflammatory drugs. Corticosteroids may be used for short periods in treating certain rare kinds of severe back pain.

Surgery

Very few people with back pain can be helped by surgery; most can be treated effectively in other ways. A herniated disc may require surgery if pain is prolonged or if the disc has produced nerve damage. Most disc problems can be treated successfully with exercise, rest, and medication. When needed, surgical operations on the back are done either by orthopedic surgeons or neurosurgeons.

Treating Emotional Stresses

Back pain is often related to emotional upsets, especially in people with chronic or repeated back pain. For this reason, many people with back pain benefit from talking openly with their families, friends, and doctors about their concerns and stresses. Emotional strain can also cause a loss of sleep, which may contribute to back pain.

Doctors and therapists often recommend that a person with chronic back pain visit with a social worker, psychologist, psychiatrist, or person at a family service agency. Visits with such professionals can help such people understand and cope with the sources of stress and emotional upset that may contribute to their back pain.

THE FUTURE

Back pain for most people eventually goes away. By following their treatment programs closely, they can shorten their periods of discomfort. They can also continue to lead their lives as usual, making only minor adjustments in their activities and workplaces, and learning better ways in which to use their backs.

The majority of people with back pain don't need to continue their medication for more than three or four weeks, but they may need to continue exercising throughout their lives to keep their back muscles strong and prevent the pain from returning.

Recently, scientists have increased their search for the causes of back pain, paying close attention to work-related causes. They have found, for example, that jobs requiring a lot of lifting, especially when a twisting motion is involved, create many back pain problems. By measuring the strength of workers hired for certain jobs requiring lifting and comparing this to the physical demands of a particular job, researchers have found that back pain is more common in people who have been matched to a job that exceeds their capability. This information is now being used to develop ways of reducing the amount of back pain caused by work-related tasks. By matching strength scores to job scores the risk of back pain in workers should be reduced.

Other investigators are examining the uses of the CAT scan for finding some of the causes of back pain. This kind of examination can locate the cause of back pain induced by a narrowing of the openings through which the spinal cord passes in the vertebrae, which is one cause of such pain.

CHAPTER TWENTY-SIX

Where Do We Go From Here?

The field of rheumatology has come a long way in a short time. Before the 1940s, many of the diseases that are now recognized as rheumatic diseases had not yet been clearly identified and could not be distinguished from each other. Most of the drugs currently used in treating rheumatic diseases either had not been invented, were not used as they are today in treating these diseases, or were still experimental. The major surgical procedures that have been so helpful to many people with severe rheumatic diseases had yet to be developed and refined. Few rheumatologists existed.

Before the present generation, the major discoveries about how the immune system works and how it malfunctions in different rheumatic diseases had not been made. Compared with what is now known, almost nothing was understood of the complex events of inflammation, nor was the role of genetics in the development of some forms arthritis appreciated.

One of the consequences of this situation was that many people who had severe rheumatoid arthritis were consigned to bed and totally crippled, which is much less common today. People with gout had repeated attacks that eventually crippled them, and no treatment could prevent this outcome.

Today, most people with rheumatic diseases can live far better than they would have in the previous generation. Many are able to function almost normally and participate in work and social activities with minimum disruption. People who have developed one of the rare, potentially fatal rheumatic diseases are surviving at much higher rates than they did only a few decades ago.

The Arthritis Foundation, which was founded in 1948, deserves some of the credit for these advances. As the only non-profit, voluntary health organization completely dedicated to finding the causes, ways of preventing, and cures for the different rheumatic diseases, it has helped bring about many of these welcome advances in research and treatment.

Joined with the Arthritis Foundation in its work are the medical professionals specializing in rheumatic diseases. The world's largest professional society of rheumatologists, the American Rheumatism Association, founded in 1934, has provided leadership in the study and control of rheumatic diseases for over fifty years. The Arthritis Health Professions Association—formed by nurses, physical and occupational therapists, medical social workers, and others—works to overcome the shortage of specialized health workers in rheumatic disease. The largest supporter of arthritis research in the United States is the U.S. government-sponsored National Institutes of Health (NIH). One of its institutes, the National Institute of Arthritis, Diabetes and Digestive and Kidney Disease, spends over forty-five million dollars a year on arthritis research. Other institutes of NIH contribute another fifteen million for this purpose. The amount spent on arthritis research, however, is many times less per patient than that spent on other serious health problems such as cancer and heart disease.

The Arthritis Foundation has sponsored research in many promising areas of rheumatic disease, and continues to do so. It provides grants to selected centers for arthritis care, research, and training. It provides training for physicians, scientists, and allied health professionals who intend to make careers in the field of rheumatic disease. At the chapter level, it provides support for individual research projects aimed at improving the diagnosis and treatment of the rheumatic diseases and furthering the knowledge of the underlying processes that cause these disorders.

The major emphases of the Arthritis Foundation's research program are on identifying causative factors involved in arthritis, with a view toward their eventual control and to train young scientists entering this field. Even in the absence of sufficient knowledge about arthritis, however, much can be learned about more effective ways of applying those treatments that are currently available for it. Since the future of rheumatic disease

259

research depends on attracting bright and energetic individuals into the field, research training is a major part of the continuing program.

Until solutions to all of the rheumatic diseases are found, the Arthritis Foundation will continue to provide services for people affected with these diseases, and is working to make the public aware that arthritis and related conditions are serious and painful. The seventy-one chapters and divisions of the Foundation reach into communities across the United States to offer information and services and to educate communities about ways of alleviating the effects of rheumatic disease.

Many Arthritis Foundation chapters have support groups to encourage people with arthritis-related diseases to share their therapies, solutions to common problems, and personal support. The Foundation's service programs include self-help courses, exercise classes, support groups, equipment loans, and referral to medical and community resources. The chapters welcome new members seeking help or offering their services as volunteers. Addresses are current as of September, 1984.

ARTHRITIS FOUNDATION
  HEADQUARTERS
1314 Spring Street, NW
Atlanta, GA 30309
Tel: (404) 872-7100

ALABAMA CHAPTER
13 Office Park Circle,
  Room 14
Birmingham, Alabama 35223
Tel: (205) 870-4700

SOUTH ALABAMA
  CHAPTER
304 Little Flower Avenue
Mobile, Alabama 36606
Tel: (205) 471-1725

CENTRAL ARIZONA
  CHAPTER
711 East Missouri,
  Suite A-116
Phoenix, Arizona 85014
Tel: (602) 264-7679

SOUTHERN ARIZONA
  CHAPTER
4520 East Grant Road
Tucson, Arizona 85712
Tel: (602) 326-2811

ARKANSAS CHAPTER
6213 Lee Avenue
Little Rock, Arkansas 72205
Tel: (501) 664-7242

NORTHEASTERN
  CALIFORNIA DIVISION
2422 Arden Way, Suite A-28
Sacramento, California 95825
(916) 921-5533

NORTHERN CALIFORNIA
  CHAPTER
203 Willow Street,
  Suite 201
San Francisco, CA 94109
(415) 673-6882

SAN DIEGO AREA
  CHAPTER
6154 Mission Gorge Road,
  Suite 110
San Diego, California 92120
Tel: (619) 280-0304

SOUTHERN CALIFORNIA
  CHAPTER
4311 Wilshire Boulevard
Los Angeles, California 90010
Tel: (213) 938-6111

ROCKY MOUNTAIN
  CHAPTER
234 Columbine Street,
  Suite 210
P.O. Box 6919
Denver, Colorado 80206
Tel: (303) 399-5065

CONNECTICUT CHAPTER
370 Silas Deane Highway
Wethersfield, Connecticut
  06109
Tel: (203) 563-1177

DELAWARE CHAPTER
234 Philadelphia Pike, Suite 1
Wilmington, Delaware 19809
Tel: (302) 764-8254

METROPOLITAN
  WASHINGTON
  CHAPTER
1901 Fort Myer Drive,
  Suite 507
Arlington, Virginia 22209
Tel: (703) 276-7555

FLORIDA CHAPTER
3205 Manatee Avenue, West
Bradenton, Florida 33505
Tel: (813) 748-1300

GEORGIA CHAPTER
1340 Spring Street,
  Suite 103
Atlanta, Georgia 30309
Tel: (404) 873-3240
Toll Free: 1-800-282-7023
  (for Georgia residents only)

HAWAII CHAPTER
200 North Vineyard, Suite 503
Honolulu, Hawaii 96817
Tel: (808) 523-7561

IDAHO CHAPTER
700 Robbins Road, Suite 1
Boise, Idaho 83702
Tel: (208) 344-7102

CENTRAL ILLINOIS
  CHAPTER
320 East Armstrong Avenue,
  Room 102
Peoria, Illinois 61603
Tel: (309) 672-6337

ILLINOIS CHAPTER
79 West Monroe, Suite 1120
Chicago, Illinois 60603
Tel: (312) 782-1367

INDIANA CHAPTER
1010 East 86th Street
Indianapolis, Indiana 46240
Tel: (317) 844-3341

261

IOWA CHAPTER
1501 Ingersoll Avenue,
    Suite 101
Des Moines, Iowa 50309
Tel: (515) 243-6259

KANSAS CHAPTER
1602 East Waterman
Wichita, Kansas 67211
Tel: (316) 263-0116

KENTUCKY CHAPTER
1381 Bardstown Road
Louisville, Kentucky 40204
Tel: (502) 459-6400

LOUISIANA CHAPTER
4700 Dryades
New Orleans, Louisiana
    70115
Tel: (504) 897-1338

MAINE CHAPTER
37 Mill Street
Brunswick, Maine 04011
Tel: (207) 729-4453

MARYLAND CHAPTER
12 West 25th Street
Baltimore, Maryland 21218
Tel: (301) 366-0923

MASSACHUSETTS
    CHAPTER
The Parker Building
124 Watertown Street
Watertown, Massachusetts
    02171
Tel: (617) 926-2900

MICHIGAN CHAPTER
23999 Northwestern Highway,
    Suite 210
Southfield, Michigan 48075
Tel: (313) 561-9096

MINNESOTA CHAPTER
122 West Franklin, Suite 440
Minneapolis, Minnesota
    55404
Tel: (612) 874-1201

MISSISSIPPI CHAPTER
6055 Ridgewood Road
Jackson, Mississippi 39211
Tel: (601) 956-3371

EASTERN MISSOURI
    CHAPTER
7315 Manchester
St. Louis, Missouri 63143
Tel: (314) 644-3488

WESTERN MISSOURI—
    GREATER KANSAS
    CITY CHAPTER
8301 State Line, Suite 117
Kansas City, Missouri 64114
Tel: (816) 361-7002

MONTANA CHAPTER
2 Polly Drive
P.O. Box 20994
Billings, Montana 59101
Tel: (406) 248-7602

NEBRASKA CHAPTER
2229 N. 91st Court, #33
Omaha, Nebraska 68134
Tel: (402) 558-2400

NEVADA DIVISION
3160 South Valley
View Boulevard, Suite 107A
Las Vegas, Nevada 89102
Tel: (702) 367-1626

NEW HAMPSHIRE
CHAPTER
P.O. Box 369
35 Pleasant Street
Concord, New Hampshire
03301
Tel: (603)224-9322

NEW JERSEY CHAPTER
15 Prospect Lane
Colonia, New Jersey 07067
Tel: (201)388-0744

NEW MEXICO CHAPTER
5112 Grand Avenue, NE
Albuquerque, New Mexico
87108
Tel: (505)265-1545

CENTRAL NEW YORK
CHAPTER
505 East Fayette Street,
2nd Floor
Syracuse, New York 13202
Tel: (315)422-8174

GENESEE VALLEY
CHAPTER
973 East Avenue
Rochester, New York 14607
Tel: (716)271-3540

LONG ISLAND DIVISION
501 Walt Whitman Road
Melville, New York 11747
Tel: (516)427-8272

NEW YORK CHAPTER
115 East 18th Street
New York, New York 10003
Tel: (212)477-8310

NORTHEASTERN NEW
YORK CHAPTER
1237 Central Avenue
Albany, New York 12205
Tel: (518)459-5082

WESTERN NEW YORK
CHAPTER
1370 Niagara Falls Boulevard
Tonawanda, New York 14150
Tel: (716)837-8600

NORTH CAROLINA
DIVISION
3115 Guess Road
Durham, North Carolina
27705
Tel: (919) 477-0286

DAKOTA CHAPTER
1402 North 39th Street
Fargo, North Dakota 58102
Tel: (701)282-3653

CENTRAL OHIO
CHAPTER
2501 North Star Road
Columbus, Ohio 43221
Tel: (614)488-0777

NORTHEASTERN OHIO
CHAPTER
11416 Bellflower Road
Cleveland, Ohio 44106
Tel: (216)791-1310

NORTHWESTERN OHIO
CHAPTER
4447 Talmadge Road
Toledo, Ohio 43623
Tel: (419)473-3349

SOUTHWESTERN OHIO
CHAPTER
2400 Reading Road
Cincinnati, Ohio 45202
Tel: (513)721-1027

EASTERN OKLAHOMA
CHAPTER
2816 East 51st Street,
Suite 120
Tulsa, Oklahoma 74105
Tel: (918)743-4526

OKLAHOMA CHAPTER
3313 Classen Boulevard,
Suite 101
Oklahoma City, Oklahoma
73118
Tel: (405)521-0066

OREGON CHAPTER
Barbur Boulevard Plaza
4445 SW Barbur Boulevard
Portland, Oregon 97201
Tel: (503)222-7246

CENTRAL
PENNSYLVANIA
CHAPTER
P.O. Box 668
2019 Chestnut Street
Camp Hill, Pennsylvania
17011
Tel: (717)763-0900

EASTERN
PENNSYLVANIA
CHAPTER
311 South Juniper Street,
Suite 201
Philadelphia, Pennsylvania
19107
Tel: (215)735-5272

WESTERN
PENNSYLVANIA
CHAPTER
2201 Clark Building
Pittsburgh, Pennsylvania
15222
Tel: (412)566-1645

RHODE ISLAND
CHAPTER
850 Waterman Avenue
East Providence, Rhode
Island 02914
Tel: (401)434-5792

SOUTH CAROLINA
CHAPTER
1802 Sumter Street
Columbia, South Carolina
29201
Tel: (803)254-6702

MIDDLE-EAST
TENNESSEE DIVISION
210 25th Ave. N. Room 1202
Nashville, Tennessee 37203
Tel: (615)329-3431

WEST TENNESSEE
CHAPTER
2600 Poplar Avenue,
Suite 200
Memphis, Tennessee 38112
Tel: (901)452-4482

NORTH TEXAS
CHAPTER
6300 Harry Hines Boulevard,
Suite 211
Exchange Park
Treadway Plaza
Dallas, Texas 75235-5207
Tel: (214) 956-7771

264

NORTHWEST TEXAS
CHAPTER
3145 McCart Avenue
Fort Worth, Texas 76110
Tel: (817)926-7733

SOUTH CENTRAL
TEXAS CHAPTER
503 South Main Street
San Antonio, Texas 78204
Tel: (512)224-4857

TEXAS GULF COAST
CHAPTER
9111—A Katy Freeway
Houston, Texas 77024
Tel: (713) 468-6572

WEST TEXAS CHAPTER
2317 34th Street
Lubbock, Texas 79411
Tel: (806)793-3273

UTAH CHAPTER
1733 South 1100 East
Salt Lake City, Utah 84105
Tel: (801) 486-4993

VERMONT CHAPTER
Richardson Place,
   Suite 2E
Church Street
Burlington, Vermont 05402
Tel: (802)864-4988

VIRGINIA CHAPTER
1900 Byrd Avenue, Suite 100
P.O. Box 6772
Richmond, Virginia 23230
Tel: (804)282-5491

WESTERN WASHINGTON
CHAPTER
726 Broadway, Suite 103
Seattle, Washington 98122
Tel: (206)324-9940

WEST VIRGINIA
CHAPTER
440 Fourth Avenue
P.O. Box 8473
South Charleston, West
   Virginia 25303
Tel: (304)744-3042

WISCONSIN CHAPTER
1442 North Farwell Avenue,
   Suite 508
Milwaukee, Wisconsin 53202
Tel: (414)276-0490
Toll Free: 1-800-242-9945

Helpful Agencies and Organizations

ACTION FOR CHILD TRANSPORTATION SAFETY, INC.
400 Central Park West, #15P
New York, NY 10025

AMERICAN ASSOCIATION FOR RETIRED PERSONS (AARP)
National Headquarters
1909 K Street, NW
Washington, DC 20049

AMERICAN FOUNDATION FOR THE BLIND
15 West 16th Street
New York, NY 10011

AMERICAN OCCUPATIONAL THERAPY ASSOCIATION
6000 Executive Boulevard
Rockville, MD 20852

AMERICAN JUVENILE ARTHRITIS ORGANIZATION
1314 Spring Street, NW
Atlanta, GA 30309

AMERICAN PHYSICAL THERAPY ASSOCIATION
1156 15th Street, NW
Washington, DC 20006

ARCHITECTURAL AND TRANSPORTATION BARRIERS
COMPLIANCE BOARD
330 C Street, SW
Washington, DC 20201

ARTHRITIS FOUNDATION
1314 Spring Street, NW
Atlanta, GA 30309

THE ARTHRITIS SOCIETY
920 Yonge Street
Suite 420
Toronto M4Y 357, Ontario
Canada

DIVISION OF VOCATIONAL REHABILITATION
(Check telephone book for regional office in your county seat.)

INDEPENDENT LIVING FOR THE DISABLED OFFICE
HUD
7th and D Streets, SW
Washington, DC 20410

INTERIOR DEPARTMENT
Washington, DC 20240
(Information on access to federal recreation areas.)

INTERNATIONAL REHABILITATION FILM REVIEW
LIBRARY
20 West 40th Street
New York, NY 10018

MOSS REHABILITATION HOSPITAL
Travel Information Center
12th Street and Tabor Road
Philadelphia, PA 19141

NATIONAL ASSOCIATION OF THE PHYSICALLY
HANDICAPPED
2 Meetinghouse Road
Merrimack, NH 03054

NATIONAL CENTER FOR A BARRIER-FREE
ENVIRONMENT
Seventh and Florida, NE
Washington, DC 20002

NATIONAL EASTER SEAL SOCIETY FOR CRIPPLED
CHILDREN & ADULTS
2023 West Ogden Avenue
Chicago, IL 60612

NATIONAL INFORMATION CENTER FOR THE
HANDICAPPED
P.O. Box 1492
Washington, DC 20013

NATIONAL INSTITUTE OF ARTHRITIS, DIABETES AND
DIGESTIVE AND KIDNEY DISEASES
Bethesda, MD 20014

NATIONAL LEAGUE FOR NURSING
10 Columbus Circle
New York, NY 10019

NATIONAL LIBRARY SERVICE FOR THE BLIND AND
PHYSICALLY HANDICAPPED
Washington, DC 20540

NATIONAL SAFETY COUNCIL
Dept. H.P.O., Box 11171
Chicago, IL 60611

NATIONAL SOCIETY FOR THE PREVENTION OF
BLINDNESS
79 Madison Avenue
New York, NY 10016

OFFICE OF CONSUMER SERVICES
U.S. Department of Health and Human Services
Washington, DC 20201

PEOPLE-TO-PEOPLE COMMITTEE FOR THE
HANDICAPPED
1028 Connecticut Avenue, NW
Washington, DC 20036

PHYSICIANS FOR AUTOMOTIVE SAFETY
50 Union Avenue
Irvington, NJ 07111

PRESIDENT'S COMMITTEE ON EMPLOYMENT OF
THE HANDICAPPED
Washington, DC 20210

PUBLIC AFFAIRS PAMPHLETS
381 Park Avenue
New York, NY 10016
(Catalog of helpful publications)

REHABILITATION INTERNATIONAL
20 West 40th Street
New York, NY 10018
(Publications and films)

REHABILITATION SERVICES ADMINISTRATION
Department of Health and Human Services
Washington, DC 20201

SISTER KENNY INSTITUTE
A/V Publication Department #266
27th at Chicago Avenue
Minneapolis, MN 55407

URBAN MASS TRANSPORTATION ADMINISTRATION
Washington, DC 20420

U.S. SOCIAL SECURITY ADMINISTRATION
Division of Disability Operations
6401 Security Boulevard
Baltimore, MD 21235

Suggested Reading

ARTHRITIS FOUNDATION PUBLICATIONS

Medical Information Series Pamphlets

Ankylosing Spondylitis
Arthritis in Children
Back Pain
Bursitis, Tendinitis & Related Conditions
Fibrositis
Gout
Infectious Arthritis
Osteoarthritis
Polymyalgia Rheumatica
Polymyositis/Dermatomyositis
Pseudogout
Psoriatic Arthritis
Reiter's Syndrome
Rheumatoid Arthritis
Scleroderma
Systemic Lupus Erythematosus

General Pamphlets

Arthritis—The Basic Facts
Aspirin and Related Medications
Gold Treatment
Diet and Nutrition
Inflammation—Unlocking the Mystery

Living and Loving
Practical Information
Quackery and Unproven Remedies
Surgery
Taking Charge: Learning to Live with Arthritis

Manuals

Overcoming Rheumatoid Arthritis
Self-Help Manual for Patients with Arthritis

Periodicals

ACCD Action. American Coalition of Citizens with Disabilities, 1346 Connecticut Avenue, NW, Washington, DC 20036. Monthly, $5 year.

Accent on Living, P.O. Box 700, Bloomington, IL 61701. Quarterly, $4 per year.

Amicus, National Center for Law and the Handicapped, Inc., 1235 North Eddy Street, South Bend, IN 46617. Free.

Arise: A New Voice for the Nation's Handicapped People, 55 West Park Avenue, New Haven, CT 06511. 10 issues per year, $5.00 from 376 Bay 44th Street, Brooklyn, NY 11214.

Closer Look, National Information Center for the Handicapped, P.O. Box 1492, Washington, DC 20013. Free information on topics of interest to persons with disabilities.

COPH Bulletin, National Congress of Organizations of the Physically Handicapped, Apt. 203, 2040 Highland Avenue, Birmingham, AL 35205. Quarterly, $2 per year.

Encore, National Library Service for the Blind and Physically Handicapped, Library of Congress, Washington, DC 20540. Bimonthly recording for Talking Books readers of selections from publications for the disabled. Available on free loan from your regional library.

Disabled USA, The President's Committee on Employment of the Handicapped, Washington, D.C. 20210. Free.

Informer, Office of Human Development, Rehabilitation Services Administration, Department of Health and Human Services, Washington, DC 20201. Free.

Mainstream: Magazine of the Able-Disabled, 861 Sixth Avenue, Suite 610, San Diego, CA 92101. Monthly, $5.00 per year.

National Hookup, P.O. Box 878, Adelanto, CA 92301. Monthly, $3 per year.

Paraplegia Life, National Paraplegia Foundation, 333 North Michigan Avenue, Chicago, IL 60601. Bimonthly, $5 membership.

Paraplegia News, 935 Coastline Drive, Seal Beach, CA 90740. Monthly, $4.50 per year.

Rehabilitation Gazette, International Journal and Information Service for the Disabled, 4502 Maryland Avenue, St. Louis, MO 63108. Annual, $3 disabled, $5 nondisabled. (Also available on cassette or tape.)

Books

Blau, Sheldon, M.D., and Dodi Schultz. *Arthritis.* Garden City, NY: Doubleday, 1973.

Bruck, Lilly. *Access: The Guide to a Better Life for Disabled Americans.* New York: Random House, 1978.

Engleman, Ephraim P., M.D., and Milton Silverman, Ph.D. *The Arthritis Book.* Sausalito, CA: Painter Hopkins, 1979.

Fries, James F., M.D. *Arthritis.* Reading, MA: Addison-Wesley, 1980.

Hale, Glorya, ed. *The Source Book for the Disabled.* New York: Bantam Books, 1979.

Healey, Louis A., M.D., Kenneth Wilske, M.D., and Bob Hansen. *Beyond the Copper Bracelet.* 2nd ed. Bowie, MD: The Charles Press, 1977.

Johnson, G. Timothy, M.D. *Coping with Arthritis.* New York: Newspaperbooks, 1977.

Lorig, Kate, R.N., Dr. P.H., and James F. Fries, M.D. *The Arthritis Helpbook.* Reading, MA: Addison-Wesley, 1980.

Lunt, Suzanne. *A Handbook for the Disabled: Ideas & Inventions for Easier Living.* New York: Charles Scribner's Sons, 1982.

Glossary

ALDOLASE—an enzyme found in muscles; it spills over into the blood in certain rheumatic diseases.

ANA—see antinuclear antibodies.

ANKYLOSING SPONDYLITIS—a disease causing inflammation of the joints of the spine that can cause the bones to fuse, or grow together.

ANTIBODIES—proteins in the blood that combine with specific foreign antigens. This combination sets off an immune reaction designed to rid the body of the antigens.

ANTIGEN—a foreign substance whose presence stimulates the immune system.

ANTIMALARIAL DRUGS—slow-acting drugs related to quinine and originally used to treat malaria; now sometimes used also in rheumatoid arthritis, systemic lupus, and discoid lupus.

ANTINUCLEAR ANTIBODIES (ANA)—a group of abnormal antibodies found in most people with lupus and scleroderma. Also found in some people with juvenile arthritis and rheumatoid arthritis. ANAs combine with the nucleus of cells.

ARTERITIS—inflammation of an artery.

ARTHRITIS—inflammation of a joint.

ARTHRODESIS—an operation in which the bones at a joint are fused together and the joint is locked in place.

ARTHROGRAM—the photographic image produced through arthrography.

ARTHROGRAPHY—an X-ray method in which a dye is injected into a joint, an X-ray is taken, and the image reveals whether there is damage to cartilage and other tissue.

ARTHROPLASTY—the rebuilding of damaged joints by resurfacing the ends of bones or the replacement of an entire joint with an artificial joint.

ARTHROSCOPY—a minor surgical procedure in which the physician inserts an instrument like a periscope into the joint and examines joint tissues; some surgery can be performed through the arthroscope.

AUTOANTIBODIES—abnormal antibodies directed against parts of a person's own body rather than against invading antigens.

AUTOIMMUNE DISEASE—a disease in which the immune system malfunctions and attacks tissues of the body, causing tissue injury and inflammation.

AZATHIOPRINE—one of the cytotoxic drugs used in treating rheumatoid arthritis, lupus, and some other rheumatic diseases.

B CELLS—see B lymphocytes.

BIOPSY—the removal of tissue for later examination with a microscope.

B LYMPHOCYTES—specialized lymphocytes that develop into plasma cells which produce antibodies.

BOUCHARD'S NODES—bony growths in the middle of the fingers; associated with osteoarthritis.

BURSAE—small, fluid-filled sacs found near joints between the muscles, bones, ligaments, and tendons; they help absorb shocks and reduce friction.

BURSITIS—inflammation of a bursa.

CALCIUM PYROPHOSPHATE DIHYDRATE CRYSTAL DEPOSITION DISEASE (CPPD DISEASE)—a chronic rheumatic disease in which unusual calcium crystals are deposited in joints; sometimes called pseudogout or chondrocalcinosis.

CARTILAGE—a rubbery material that cushions the ends of the bones and absorbs shock.

CAT SCAN—see computerized axial tomography.

CHRONIC DISEASE—a disease that lasts for many years or perhaps a lifetime.

COLLAGEN—the major structural protein of connective tissue.

COMPLEMENT SYSTEM—a group of proteins that circulate in the blood; they are involved in immune reactions and promote inflammation and cause immune complexes to be destroyed by scavenger cells.

COMPLETE BLOOD COUNT—diagnostic tests showing the numbers of different cellular components of the blood, such as white blood cells, red blood cells, and platelets.

COMPUTERIZED AXIAL TOMOGRAPHY—a special X-ray technique in which a computer helps create cross-sectional views of portions of the body.

CONNECTIVE TISSUE—a type of supportive tissue that is diffusely distributed throughout the body; helps form membranes to hold internal organs in place, cartilage, muscles, tendons, ligaments, and skin.

CONTRACTURE—see flexion contracture.

CORTICOSTEROIDS—a group of drugs related to the natural hormones cortisone and hydrocortisone; potent drugs that quickly reduce pain and inflammation but carry a risk of serious side effects.

CPPD DISEASE—see calcium pyrophosphate dihydrate crystal deposition (CPPD) disease.

CREATINE PHOSPHOKINASE (CPK)—an enzyme found in muscles; it spills over into the blood in certain diseases of muscles.

CREATININE TEST—a diagnostic test that measures how much creatinine—a normal waste product of the body—is present in the blood; the test indicates how well the kidneys are functioning.

CRYOTHERAPY—the use of cold treatments to relieve pain.

CYCLOPHOSPHAMIDE—one of the cytotoxic drugs used in certain serious rheumatic diseases.

CYTOTOXIC DRUGS—potent, slow-acting drugs primarily used to treat cancer and in people who receive organ transplants; sometimes used for serious rheumatoid arthritis, psoriatic arthritis, systemic lupus, vasculitis, and polymyositis.

DERMATOMYOSITIS—a rheumatic disease that causes weakness and inflammation of certain muscles, possible joint inflammation, and skin rashes.

DISCOID LUPUS—a form of lupus that affects only the skin.

DISEASE-MODIFYING DRUGS—see slow-acting drugs.

ELECTROMYOGRAM—a diagnostic test of muscle function; measures the electrical pattern generated by muscles.

EMG—see electromyogram.

ERYTHROCYTE SEDIMENTATION RATE—a diagnostic test that measures how fast red blood cells fall to the bottom of a tube; it indicates presence and degree of inflammation.

ESR—see erythrocyte sedimentation rate.

FIBROMYALGIA—see fibrositis.

FIBROSITIS—a condition in which there is generalized pain in the muscles, ligaments, and tendons without damage to any of these structures.

FLARE-UP—a period during which disease symptoms reappear or become worse.

FLEXION CONTRACTURE—the condition in which a joint is stuck in the bent position; it is often preventable with daily stretching exercises.

FUSION (OF BONES)—see arthrodesis.

GENES—units of DNA—the chemical blueprints of inheritance—that instruct cells to make proteins to perform the body's functions.

GENETIC MARKER—a specific type of body chemical often found on tissue cells; similar to a blood type, that is passed on from one generation to the next in the genes; some genetic markers are linked with certain rheumatic diseases.

GIANT-CELL ARTERITIS—an illness, often associated with poly-myalgia rheumatica, that causes certain arteries to become inflamed.

GOLD TREATMENT—a type of slow-acting drug treatment some-times used for rheumatoid arthritis, juvenile arthritis, and psoriatic arthritis.

GOUT—a form of arthritis in which the body builds up too much uric acid; uric acid crystals then collect in joints and cause painful attacks.

GRANULOCYTES—the most prevalent white cells in the blood; they respond quickly to any foreign substance, immune com-plex, or injury by migrating into the area and attacking the offending agent.

HEBERDEN'S NODES—bony growths in the finger joints closest to the nails; associated with osteoarthritis.

"HELPER" T LYMPHOCYTE—a certain kind of T lymphocyte that helps activate B lymphocytes to produce antibodies.

HLA—see human leukocyte antigens.

HLA-B27—a genetic marker associated with an increased risk of developing ankylosing spondylitis or Reiter's syndrome.

HLA-DR4—a genetic marker associated with an increased risk of developing rheumatoid arthritis.

HUMAN LEUKOCYTE ANTIGENS (HLA)—specific genetic markers of great interest to rheumatic disease experts; several are related to an increased tendency to develop certain rheu-matic diseases.

HYPERURICEMIA—a condition in which uric acid levels in the blood are elevated; leads to gout in some people.

IMMUNE COMPLEX—the combination of an antibody with its antigen.

IMMUNE SYSTEM—the body's natural defense system against in-jury or infection.

IMMUNOLOGY—the study of the functions and malfunctions of the immune system.

IMMUNOSUPPRESSANT—see cytotoxic drugs.

IMMUNOSUPPRESSIVE DRUGS—see cytotoxic drugs.

INFECTIOUS ARTHRITIS—arthritis that develops as a result of an infection of the joint by a bacterium, virus, or fungus.

INFLAMMATION—a reaction of the body to injury or disease, causing pain, swelling, redness, warmth, and sometimes loss of motion in the area affected.

ISOMETRIC EXERCISE—an exercise that involves no joint movement but is designed to improve muscle strength.

JOINT—any place in the body where two bones come together.

JOINT ASPIRATION—the removal of joint fluid.

JRA—juvenile rheumatoid arthritis; see juvenile arthritis.

JUVENILE ARTHRITIS—a general term that refers to several kinds of arthritis that occur in children; also called juvenile rheumatoid arthritis.

LEUKOTRIENES—natural chemicals in the body that are very potent producers of inflammation.

LIGAMENT—a strong cordlike structure that connects bones to other bones.

LUPUS—see systemic lupus erythematosus.

LYME DISEASE—a form of infectious arthritis spread by the bite of a tick that is carrying a certain spirochete (a type of bacterium).

LYMPH NODES—small, compact structures of the immune system found in many areas of the body; the lymph nodes are where the disease-fighting lymphocytes are made.

LYMPHOCYTES—specialized white blood cells that help the immune system fight off disease; two major categories are T lymphocytes and B lymphocytes.

MACROPHAGE—specialized white blood cells that recognize and present antigens to lymphocytes and help initiate the immune response against the antigens.

METHOTREXATE—one of the cytotoxic drugs.

MUSCULAR RHEUMATISM—see fibrositis.

MUSCULOSKELETAL PAIN SYNDROME—see fibrositis.

MYELOGRAM—a special X-ray procedure in which a dye is injected into the spinal canal, an X-ray is taken, and the resulting image reveals whether any intervertebral discs have bulged and are pressing on nerves.

MYOSITIS—a term referring to polymyositis and dermatomyositis.

NONARTICULAR RHEUMATISM—see fibrositis.

NONSTEROIDAL ANTI-INFLAMMATORY DRUGS—the most commonly used category of drugs for arthritis; they reduce pain and inflammation.

NSAIDS—see nonsteroidal anti-inflammatory drugs.

OCCUPATIONAL THERAPIST—a health professional trained to help people improve efficiency in completing daily tasks at home or work; he or she demonstrates the use of assistive devices and makes aids such as splints for resting joints and preventing deformity.

OPHTHALMOLOGIST—a medical doctor who specializes in eye care.

ORTHOPEDIC SURGEON—a physician specializing in surgery of the musculoskeletal system (bones, joints, and muscles).

OSTEOARTHRITIS—the most common form of arthritis; it involves the chronic breakdown of cartilage in the affected joints.

OSTEOPHYTES—small bony growths; present in people with osteoarthritis.

OSTEOTOMY—the surgical correction of a joint deformity by cutting, then resetting a bone in the proper alignment.

PANNUS—in rheumatoid arthritis, a destructive growth of thickened, inflamed synovial membrane that penetrates and damages the bone and cartilage of the joint.

PAUCIARTICULAR JUVENILE RHEUMATOID ARTHRITIS —a form of juvenile arthritis that affects only one or a few joints.

PENICILLAMINE—one of the slow-acting drugs; it is sometimes used in serious rheumatoid arthritis.

PHYSIATRIST—a medical doctor specializing in physical medicine and rehabilitation.

PHYSICAL THERAPIST—a health professional who is trained to assist people in carrying out therapeutic exercises and using techniques to relieve pain.

PLACEBO—an inactive, harmless preparation given as a medicine to a person who is acting as a control in testing the effectiveness of another, active substance.

PLACEBO EFFECT—temporary improvement in a person's health after he or she takes a harmless, inactive substance with the belief that it will cause improvement; the effect shows the power of the mind over the body.

PLASMAPHERESIS—an experimental treatment in which plasma is removed from the blood, "cleansed" of certain substances, and returned to the body.

PLATELETS—small, round disc-like cells in the blood that are involved in the clotting process.

POLYARTICULAR JUVENILE RHEUMATOID ARTHRITIS— a form of juvenile arthritis in which many joints are affected.

POLYMORPHONUCLEAR LEUKOCYTES—see granulocytes.

POLYMYALGIA RHEUMATICA—a rheumatic disease that causes pain and stiffness in certain groups of muscles.

POLYMYOSITIS—a rheumatic disease causing weakness and inflammation of muscles and sometimes joint inflammation.

PROSTAGLANDINS—natural, hormonelike chemicals that are involved in inflammation; some prostaglandins increase inflammation and others slow it down.

PROTEOGLYCAN—a large molecule consisting of proteins and sugars; a major component of cartilage.

PSEUDOGOUT—see calcium pyrophosphate dihydrate crystal deposition (CPPD) disease.

PSORIATIC ARTHRITIS—a form of arthritis that accompanies and is directly related to the skin condition known as psoriasis.

QUACKERY—the practice of overpromoting unproven products to the public for a specific use or variety of uses without enough evidence that they are safe and effective.

RANGE OF MOTION—all of the normal movements that a joint can make in different directions.

RAYNAUD'S PHENOMENON—an extreme sensitivity to cold; the fingers turn blue or very pale in response to cold.

REFERRED PAIN—pain felt at a spot different from its source.

REITER'S SYNDROME—a type of arthritis often associated with prior infections of the bowels or genito-urinary system, and associated with the genetic marker HLA-B27.

REMISSION—a period during which disease symptoms are reduced or gone.

RESECTION—the surgical removal of a tissue such as a bone or part of a bone.

RHEUMATIC DISEASES—a group of diseases that affect muscles, ligaments, tendons, joints, and sometimes other body parts.

RHEUMATISM—pain and aching in the soft tissues near joints: muscles, bursae, tendons, ligaments.

RHEUMATOID ARTHRITIS—a common and systemic type of arthritis in which the primary physical effect is inflammation in the joints.

RHEUMATOID FACTOR—an abnormal antibody often present in people with rheumatoid arthritis.

RHEUMATOLOGIST—a medical doctor specializing in the diagnosis and treatment of arthritis or other rheumatic diseases.

SCLERODERMA—a rheumatic disease of the connective tissue; it primarily affects the skin and blood vessels, but may affect many other tissues and organs.

SEDIMENTATION RATE—see erythrocyte sedimentation rate.

SLOW-ACTING DRUGS—a category of potent drugs used in some people with rheumatic diseases; these drugs include gold, penicillamine, cytotoxic drugs, and antimalarial drugs.

SOCIAL WORKER—a professional trained to counsel people to find needed services such as visiting nurses, meals-on-wheels, financial assistance, mental health programs, and so forth.

SPONDYLITIS—see ankylosing spondylitis.

STEROID DRUGS—see corticosteroids.

"SUPPRESSOR" T LYMPHOCYTE—a certain kind of T lymphocyte that slows the production of antibodies.

SYNOVECTOMY—an operation to remove diseased synovium.

SYNOVIAL FLUID—a slippery fluid found inside the joint that provides lubrication and allows for smooth, easy motion.

SYNOVIAL MEMBRANE—the lining of the inside of a joint; also called synovium.

SYNOVIUM—see synovial membrane.

SYSTEMIC DISEASE—a disease that can affect many parts of the body, not only a small area.

SYSTEMIC JUVENILE RHEUMATOID ARTHRITIS—a form of juvenile arthritis that affects numerous areas of the body, including internal organs.

SYSTEMIC LUPUS ERYTHEMATOSUS—an autoimmune rheumatic disease that often affects the skin, joints, and sometimes internal organs; it can also involve connective tissue in many parts of the body as well as blood cells.

T CELLS—see T lymphocytes.

TENDONITIS—inflammation of a tendon.

TENDON—the strong, cordlike, tapered end of a muscle that connects the muscle to a bone.

T LYMPHOCYTES—specialized lymphocytes that may react with tissue and may be involved in inflammation. Some of these also regulate the production of antibodies by B lymphocytes.

TOPHI—deposits of urate crystals that form just under the skin; they occur in gout.

TRANSAMINASE—an enzyme found in muscles; it spills over into the blood in certain rheumatic diseases.

TRIGGER POINTS—certain spots on the body that are particularly painful and tender in people with fibrositis.

URATE CRYSTALS—the crystals composed of uric acid that irritate the joints in gout.

URIC ACID—a chemical in the body that, in gout, changes into crystals and collects in the joints, causing painful attacks.

URINALYSIS—the name for a series of diagnostic tests done to determine the contents of the urine.

INDEX